RATIONING:
TALK AND ACTION IN HEALTH CARE

RATIONING: TALK AND ACTION IN HEALTH CARE

Edited by BILL NEW

Senior Research Officer, The King's Fund Policy Institute, London, UK

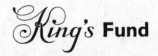

First published in 1997
by the BMJ Publishing Group, BMA House, Tavistock Square,
London WC1H 9JR
and the King's Fund, Cavendish Square, London W1M 0AN

British Library Cataloguing in Publication Data

A catalogue record for this book is available from the
British Library

ISBN 0-7279-1180-5

Contents

Section 2   "Action"

Contributors

Felix Bochner
Head, Clinical Pharmacology Unit, Royal Adelaide Hospital, Adelaide, Australia

Naomi G Burgess
Acting Director, Pharmacy Distribution Services, Royal Adelaide Hospital, Adelaide, Australia

Ruth Chadwick
Professor of Moral Philosophy, Centre for Professional Ethics, University of Central Lancashire, Preston, Lancashire, UK

Joanna Coast
Lecturer in Health Economics, Department of Social Medicine, University of Bristol, Bristol, UK

Anna Coote
Deputy Director, Institute of Public Policy Research, 30–32 Southampton Street, London, UK

A Coppel
Assistant Director, National Prescribing Centre, The Infirmary, Liverpool, UK

Roger Crisp
Fellow in Philosophy, St Anne's College, University of Oxford, Oxford, UK

Tony Culyer
Head, Department of Economics and Related Studies, University of York, Heslington, York, UK

Cam Donaldson
Professor of Economics, University of Aberdeen, Aberdeen, UK

Peter Dormer
Writer, London, UK (died December 1996)

Len Doyal
Professor of Medical Ethics, St Bartholomew's and The London School of Medicine and Dentistry, Queen Mary and Westfield College, London, UK

David Ebbs
GP, Didcot Health Centre Practice, Didcot, Oxon, UK

Josep Figueras
Regional Advisor in Health Systems Analysis, WHO Regional Office for Europe, Copenhagen, Denmark

Heather Goodare
Chair, Research Committee, UK Breast Cancer Coalition, and Counsellor in Private Practice, Horsham, West Sussex, UK

John Grimley Evans
Professor of Clinical Geratology, Nuffield Department of Clinical Medicine, The Radcliffe Infirmary, Oxford, UK

David C Hadorn
Consultant, National Advisory Committee on Health and Disability, Ministry of Health, Wellington, New Zealand

John Harris
Sir David Alliance Professor of Bioethics, Institute of Medicine, Law and Bioethics, Universities of Manchester and Liverpool, Centre for Social Ethics and Policy, Manchester, UK

Stephen Harrison
Reader in Health Policy and Politics, Nuffield Institute for Health, University of Leeds, Leeds, UK

J L Hayworth
Medical Advisor, East Lancashire Health Committee, Nelson, Lancashire, UK

Chris Heginbotham
Chief Executive, East and North Hertfordshire Health Authority, Welwyn Garden City, Hertfordshire, UK

CONTRIBUTORS

Andrew C Holmes
Senior Medical Advisor, National Advisory Committee on Health and Disability, Ministry of Health, Wellington, New Zealand

Tony Hope
Lecturer in Practice Skills and Reader in Medicine, Division of Public Health and Primary Care, Institute of Health Sciences, Oxford, UK

Rudolf Klein ·
Professorial Fellow, King's Fund Policy Institute, 11–13 Cavendish Square, London, UK

Jack Kneeshaw
Research Student, Department of Government, University of Essex, Colchester, UK

Jo Lenaghan
Research Fellow in Health Policy, Institute for Public Policy Research, 30–32 Southampton Street, London, UK

E Dean Martin
Deputy Director of Pharmacy, Clinical Pharmacology Unit, Royal Adelaide Hospital, Adelaide, Australia

Martin McKee
Professor of European Public Health, Health Services Research Unit, London School of Hygiene and Tropical Medicine, London, UK

Gary M H Misan
Executive Director, Australian Medicines Handbook Pty Ltd, Adelaide, Australia

Elizabeth Mitchell
Communications Officer, Cambridge and Huntingdon Health Authority, Fulborn Hospital, Cambridge, UK

Bill New
Senior Research Officer, The King's Fund Policy Institute, 11–13 Cavendish Square, London, UK

S Noyce
Pharmaceutical Advisor, Sefton Health Authority, Burlington House, Liverpool, UK

J C Petrie
Professor, Department of Medicine and Therapeutics, University of Aberdeen, UK

E Rous
Consultant in Public Health Medicine, Stockport Health Authority, Stockport, UK

Andrew A Somogyi
Associate Professor, Department of Clinical and Experimental Pharmacology, University of Adelaide, Adelaide, Australia

David C Thomasma
Director, Medical Humanities Program, Loyola University Chicago, Stritch School of Medicine, Maywood, IL 60153, USA

Peter Toon
General Practitioner, 206 Queensbridge Road, London, UK

Alan Williams
Professor of Economics, Centre for Health Economics, University of York, Heslington, York, UK

Acknowledgments

This book was made possible in part by a grant from the Nuffield Trust (formerly the Nuffield Provincial Hospitals Trust) which was used to commission some of the chapters included here. All the members of the RAG (see page 29 for the original signatories) contributed enormously to the production of *The rationing agenda in the NHS* and to various other aspects of the RAG's work; individual members produced some of the chapters reprinted in this book. Many thanks are due to them for their continuing support and assistance. In addition, Ann Bowling, Chris Ham and Rudolf Klein read early drafts of chapter 5 and made many valuable comments. We are also grateful to all those who responded to our *Agenda* whose comments form the basis for chapter 3.

We are grateful to *Quality in Health Care* for allowing us to reprint Len Doyal's contribution to chapter 11.

Introduction and context

1 Introduction

BILL NEW

This book derives from a continuing belief in an unpalatable truth: it is not possible to provide all the health care for everyone who could benefit from it. Wants exceed resources, and in an endless variety of ways. Clinicians' time, a new drug, staff training, extra diagnostic tests, a screening programme, medical research—all of these things, and many more, could provide additional health benefits if we devoted more resources to them. Raising expenditure can always produce *some* measurable improvement in health. But doing more becomes increasingly difficult, and squeezing out the last drops of benefit is simply unaffordable. A line has to be drawn somewhere—and the consequence is rationing.

The Rationing Agenda Group (RAG) was formed late in 1995 to promote a continuing, broad and deep debate about rationing in the National Health Service (NHS). The RAG consists of people from all parts of health care whose views on the substantive issues of rationing differ widely. Some believe in setting clear objectives and developing principles for moving towards these objectives; others would rather take a more pragmatic route, considering individual cases on their merits. Some want explicitness about why choices are made the way they are at all levels of the NHS; others worry about how this might affect confidence in the doctor–patient relationship. Many would like healthcare spending to be substantially increased; some believe we should use the resources we have more efficiently first. The RAG as a whole is united on only two points: that rationing is inevitable, and that the general public must be involved in the debate about it. In fact, a third element of consensus emerged during the course of our deliberations: the method of financing the NHS should continue to be based on general taxation. Our belief that rationing is inevitable does not imply that we wish to change the fundamental collectivist principles on which the NHS is based.

Involving the public in the debate is the long term goal. The RAG has only made the first tentative steps in this direction, but it can be easy to forget why it was an objective in the first place. Actively promoting a message that people will not be able to have all the health care that they need is at first sight highly irresponsible. Why make a difficult situation worse? Surely it would be better for the NHS to tell the public and its

3

patients only what they need to know, and avoid crossing bridges until absolutely necessary.

The RAG takes a different view: it is simply not possible to keep a well-informed and well-educated citizenry in the dark. Examples of denied care will be placed before them regularly by the media, often in melodramatic style. Without a general culture of debate about why this is happening, the result will be confusion. If the official line is to deny that rationing is inevitable, or indeed that it occurs at all, trust in those who are responsible for the NHS will continue to erode. The public are unlikely to respect an institution whose masters fail to preach what it practises.

Medical care is still shrouded in mystery, even mystique. It may not be commonly appreciated that, very often, health care can do little for us. Many treatments deliver only marginal benefits—small probabilities of success, for example, or relief of symptoms. These margins can always be extended but improvements are not priceless. By taking this debate out into the open the public will be encouraged to think about the limits of medicine, and of the costs of pursuing those limits.

In essence, the strategy is motivated by belief that frankness and honesty should pervade debates about public policy. That is the only basis on which to address the difficult task of conducting rationing more equitably and democratically. So far the RAG has pitched its thinking at the policy level as we struggled to map the agenda so that we could talk about it sensibly. In many ways this book represents the end of the RAG's first stage of work. It may not yet be of particular interest to the ordinary citizen, but we hope that a collection of the latest thought and action on rationing will nevertheless be a useful platform on which to build.

Contents

The RAG's first task was to set out all the rationing issues as an agenda, reprinted as chapter 2. This was simply designed to be a template for future work: it does not outline philosophical theories for resolving rationing dilemmas, but merely maps the dilemmas themselves. The agenda was written in the spirit of clarifying the nature of the problem; it revealed, if nothing else, that the problem is a vast one.

As part of the RAG's early work, we circulated this document to people and institutions in the NHS and policy world. We asked for reaction and suggestions; Jo Lenaghan analyses the responses in chapter 3. Most were positive, particularly on the substantive position that rationing is inevitable. Most of the respondents were not clinicians, however, and this reaction may simply reflect a managerial view of the NHS, a factor that perhaps also explains the less consensual view on how to involve the public.

Section 1 of the book deals with the theoretical policy debate—with "talk". Chris Heginbotham tackles the question of why rationing is inevitable in the NHS from his position as a purchaser in chapter 4. He concludes that it would be quite easy to spend an extra £6 billion on the NHS simply by increasing staffing levels and salaries by 10%. So even if it were possible to eliminate genuine waste in the NHS, the resulting savings pale into insignificance in the face of what it is possible to do. He also makes the point that eliminating "ineffective" services is often a disingenuous method of undertaking rationing by other means. Very few services genuinely do nothing, and many provide benefits that are intangible, delayed, uncertain or hidden—but real none the less. Attempting to call these services "ineffective" is a dangerous semantic blurring. Argue for their reduction if you wish, but do not pretend that it is not rationing.

Jack Kneeshaw reviews what we know about public opinion on rationing in chapter 5. The short answer is very little, partly because there have been few surveys and partly because the responses depend on the way in which the questions are posed. Nevertheless, apart from the shred of evidence that opinion is shifting, it still seems clear that a significant proportion of the public do not accept the inevitability of rationing. Rather more encouraging is the tentative finding that the more information and time for deliberation the public are given, the more their opinions converge towards consensus.

The following six chapters were especially commissioned by the RAG to explore some of the most important issues in more depth; the objective was not to strive for agreement at this stage but instead to reveal clearly the diversity of reasoned opinion that exists. Authors were commissioned who were known to have opposing points of view, but not all resulted in entirely polarised positions. Jo Lenaghan and Stephen Harrison, for example, both agree that some increased role for the political centre is necessary. Alan Williams and Grimley Evans, however, reveal how unreconcilable some views can be, in this case on the appropriateness of age as a rationing criterion. And Len Doyal, in his second contribution, reminds us that even unremarkable proposals such as involving the public in rationing decisions can have serious consequences, and should be subject to strict limits.

Each of these papers was originally written blind; authors were not entitled to view the piece by their "opponents" before submission. Subsequently, though, they were given the opportunity to respond to the opposing point of view, and these are appended as rejoinders to the original papers. Not all took this opportunity: absence of a rejoinder indicates satisfaction that the case cannot be improved upon and is not an editorial error!

Section 2 of the book moves from words to action: six examples of innovation in rationing practice. The first two linked papers describe a

New Zealand project to develop standardised sets of criteria for admitting patients from waiting lists for a number of elective surgical procedures. The idea is to promote a systematic assessment of priority and thereby improve accountability and efficiency. It should also improve equity by encouraging like patients to be treated equally. The second paper looks at the scheme as applied to coronary artery bypass graft surgery. The scheme is not uncontroversial—social factors such as the existence of dependants were included as relevant criteria—and is only one step on a road that could lead to a booking system replacing waiting lists altogether. But it is an example of action at the highest level, with the sanction of government.

The Swedish Government has also acted. Their Ministry of Health and Social Affairs published a report in 1995, *Priorities in health care*, and in chapter 13 Martin McKee and Josep Figueras describe how the report came to be written, the process of consultation that took place, and the principles that the report recommended should inform priority setting at all levels of the Swedish healthcare system. They emphasise how Britain could learn from this approach in its ability to provoke a national debate about rationing, and the need for an in depth and non-partisan approach for investigating the issues. The Swedes have demonstrated that broad consensus is possible on the ethical principles even during times of political conflict on other matters. Devising ethical principles does not constitute a grand solution, but neither is a grand solution necessary in order to make progress.

The third chapter in this section looks at a radical new mechanism for involving the public in rationing decisions: citizens' juries. Lenaghan and colleagues describe the experience of the first jury to be run in the UK in Cambridge and Huntingdon Health Authority. The idea of providing lay citizens with the time, space, and information to deliberate deeply about a public policy question is not new: they have run in similar formats in the USA and Germany for more than 20 years. The experiment found that the public were willing and able to grapple with difficult rationing questions, but the challenge now is to devise ways of ensuring that this (expensive) procedure can achieve real results in challenging the way public bodies make decisions. Too much public consultation is easily dismissed as window dressing.

The Asbury draft policy on the ethical use of resources, reprinted as chapter 15, is an attempt to state clearly the principles that determine how that practice uses the resources at its disposal now that it is a fundholder. The contents of the proposal provoked both admiration of the intent and scepticism of the substance—some commentators' responses are appended to the chapter. But perhaps the significant achievement for the long run is the openness with which the partners are addressing the choices that they need to make.

The licensing of a new drug, interferon-β, for the treatment of some of those who have multiple sclerosis, caused a flurry of media interest during 1996 and 1997. It is not a cure, it is expensive, and it provides only limited benefits. Some health authorities felt unable to provide specific funding for this drug, considering that other claims had greater weight. The result was a development of a patchwork of availability, with patients gaining access partly as a result of where they lived. Rous and colleagues describe the pressures that one such health authority felt as they tried to develop a strategy for managing the introduction of this drug. They did not feel able to refuse funding, but the implication, again, is that the government must take a greater lead if some semblance of equity is to be sustained.

Finally, rationing drugs in a hospital setting provides a good example of the difficulty of bridging the gap between talk and action. Bochner and colleagues describe a system that they have developed to manage the introduction of new drugs into the hospital formulary in a more systematic way. The formula they use seems complex, but the authors feel that it helps, and at least makes them more accountable. Responses from academic colleagues, particularly Donaldson, were sceptical. The use of formulae can be too rigid and may result in worse decisions than if some subjectivity remained. The original authors replied again, exasperated: surely some method has to be devised if rigour and accountability are to be improved?

This last chapter, perhaps better than all the others, emphasises where we are in the rationing debate. Fine words and sophisticated arguments are now common. Action is also well under way, in a wide variety of contexts and with much innovation. But the link between the two worlds is tenuous; very often the respective participants appear to speak different languages. Practitioners and theorists should find themselves around the same table more often, but if the UK is to emulate some of our international partners then government must take a lead. The subject is that important.

2 The rationing agenda in the NHS

BILL NEW on behalf of the Rationing Agenda Group

Preliminaries

How does rationing differ, if at all, from priority setting or resource allocation?

The terms "rationing", "priority setting", and "resource allocation" are often used interchangeably, but in some instances specific meanings are implied. These other interpretations include the following:

- "Rationing" implies exclusion or denial of a service
- "Rationing" refers to withholding, without consent, potentially beneficial treatment or to any non-market allocation of resources (this interpretation is common in the USA)
- "Priority setting" relates to services or client groups; "rationing" relates to individual cases
- "Priority setting/resource allocation" tends to entail value judgments; "rationing" tends to be more technical, based on effectiveness (or vice versa).

We believe these semantic distinctions are merely variations on the same fundamental question relating to the allocation of NHS resources. How do we choose which beneficial services should be offered to whom and which should not? The question of benefit is analysed further below. However, we consider that healthcare services that are not regarded by anyone as beneficial under any circumstances are not relevant to this topic. In short, the empirical quest to establish which medical interventions have no benefit is not a question of rationing.

In this chapter we use "rationing" as a summary term to describe this process of choosing between beneficial services. We have adopted this term because it provokes the greatest public controversy: using alternative terms does not avoid the need to address the fundamental problem clearly and coherently.

Can healthcare be delivered without rationing?

Our strategy is simply to present the issues, not take up positions on them. However, on two points we hold substantive views—that rationing is inevitable and that we need to be more explicit about the principles and issues. But is this allegedly fundamental problem really fundamental at all? If more resources were made available could this choice not be avoided altogether? Frequently suggested means of making more resources available include the following:

- Improve the efficiency with which existing services are provided
- Stop offering services that are of no proved benefit
- Redeploy resources from lower priority public services (defence is a frequently cited potential source)
- Raise taxes (that is, redeploy resources from goods and services that people buy for themselves).

We have no doubt that adopting any one or more of these strategies could ease the resource constraints faced by the healthcare system, and we could then proceed gradually to discover how far we needed to go before exhausting all the beneficial services that the NHS might provide. During this redeployment process, however, the healthcare system would be faced with deciding which of those beneficial services that it had previously chosen not to offer, now to offer (and to whom). This also requires a decision on which services still not to offer (yet). Hence providing more resources still requires the fundamental issues to be faced. The context within which they are faced will be different and the thresholds will vary but the principles that are applied will still need analysis if there is to be a well informed and responsible public debate about which are the more important new services to offer with the extra resources.

What is the range of services relevant to issues of healthcare rationing?

Typically, two ways of specifying exclusions from NHS provision are proposed. The first is on the ground of relative ineffectiveness—that is, the service does not produce enough benefit. As noted above, in the extreme case of absolutely no benefit this is not a rationing issue. However, occasionally the rationale for exclusion may be that a service produces very little or uncertain benefit or that there is a very small likelihood of success. To exclude on any of these bases would be to undertake a rationing decision, as a choice is being made between people who could benefit—if to differing degrees and with differing expectations of success.

The second way proposed to specify exclusions is on the ground of lack of relative cost effectiveness—that is, the service in question does not produce enough benefit relative to its cost when compared with other

9

services. However, it is never suggested that services with either of these characteristics are not in principle part of the business of the NHS. Indeed, if circumstances changed—for example, if technological advance made a once very expensive service much cheaper—then the provision of these services might be supported. Both "cost" and "effectiveness" are simply criteria for choosing between competing claims on resources; using them to specify packages or exclusions is the logical extension of their use as criteria for choosing between cases. Issues of this kind are discussed below.

There is, however, another basis for excluding services from the NHS. Exclusions can be simply because the type of service concerned or type of benefit it produces is not relevant to the NHS. Exclusions on this basis recognise that not everything of benefit can necessarily claim to be relevant to a healthcare system. For example, it may be more appropriate to provide a service through some other agency such as local government or the voluntary sector, or commercially by the private sector. Currently controversial services with regard to this issue include various forms of cosmetic treatment, physiotherapy for sports injuries, dentistry, eye checks and provision of spectacles, long term nursing, and infertility treatment.

There are at least two subsidiary questions: who should make the decision about what constitutes the range of relevant services (see Box 1), and what criteria are appropriate for establishing them? The following offer some possibilities for the second question:

Box 1: Categories of people who may be relevant to various rationing issues

- The general public:
  As citizens
  As taxpayers
  As potential patients
  Others?
- Patients
- Patients' families and friends
- Interest and user groups or community representatives
- Healthcare professionals—clinicians or non-clinicians
- Managers
- Central government—politicians and civil servants
- Local government—elected representatives and officers
- "Experts" in specific aspects of health and healthcare (for example, health economists, ethicists, or epidemiologists)
- Media—press and broadcast
- Industry (for example, pharmaceutical companies)
- Groups with "moral authority" (for example, clergy)
- Judiciary

- The service should constitute "health" care (rather than "social" care, for example)
- The service should display characteristics that make it unsuitable for market exchange (for example, on equity grounds)
- The service should not be appropriate to leave to the responsibility of the person who desires it.

Even if it is possible clearly to specify which services are to be included this does not mean that they will necessarily be provided to everyone who makes a claim. It will then be necessary to ask the question posed below.

Ethics

Ethical reasoning seeks principles for evaluating policies and decision making: what are right actions or good states of affairs? Equity, justice, and fairness are key ethical concepts in rationing—like patients should be treated equally and unlike patients unequally to the extent that their differences are morally relevant. The notion of efficiency as understood in the context of rationing healthcare is presented in this chapter as an ethical choice, typically concerned with maximising improvements in health for the population as a whole. Our concern with efficiency here is not in the sense of eliminating waste in the deployment of resources—that is, minimising the cost at which a given distribution of healthcare is provided—as we take this as axiomatic.

What are the objectives of the NHS, and what is the range of ethically defensible criteria for discriminating between competing claims for resources that is relevant to achieving these objectives?

If objectives are correctly specified and agreed as appropriate, then criteria relevant to achieving them must be "ethically defensible". But in the light of difficulties in achieving this specification and agreement there may remain a need to assess independently certain criteria on an ethical basis. Furthermore, there may be occasions when objectives are agreed on but there are several ways of achieving them, some of which may not be ethically defensible.

When considering the objectives of the NHS we must first try to specify the range of benefits which the NHS provides. Our concern is with "outcome" objectives—those that relate to health and other aspects of people's wellbeing—though we could focus on "structure" (facilities and resources) or "process" (volume and nature of work done).

11

There seem to be two kinds of outcome objectives: personal benefits and public benefits. Personal benefits are those that people enjoy exclusively for themselves—for example, when one person receives an improvement in health related quality of life, no one else receives this improvement as well. These sorts of benefits derive from healthcare interventions. Public benefits are those that we all enjoy at the same time without one person's enjoyment diminishing anyone else's—no one is or can be excluded. These benefits derive from the system of healthcare rather than a particular intervention. They can be enjoyed by those who may never use the healthcare system—for example, the reassurance derived from having an accident and emergency department available may benefit someone who never needs it.

Examples of these various types of benefits are listed as follows:

Personal benefits from healthcare (see Box 2)

- Mortality related
- Morbidity related
- Health related quality of life
- Composites (usually combining mortality with one of the others)
- Satisfaction
- Morally related.

Public benefits from healthcare system

- Security reassurance, "tranquillity"
- Sense of social justice
- Facilitate central control and accountability for public expenditure on healthcare.

Questions about the objectives of the NHS should be posed in terms of these benefits. Which of these benefits should be the focus of interest for the NHS? How should personal benefits be distributed, or should they simply be as large as possible? If two or more kinds of benefit are judged relevant, in what order of priority should they be placed? If they conflict how much of one should be reduced in order that another may be satisfied more fully?

Some possibilities for the objectives of the NHS might be:

- Maximising health gain (for example, maximising quality adjusted life years)

- Minimising health inequalities for geographical areas, groups, or individuals
- Improving the position of the worst off for geographical areas, groups, or individuals
- Social reassurance, stability, cohesion
- Assistance for certain disadvantaged groups
- Control of national public health expenditure
- Regulation of the delivery of care to avoid unnecessary or inappropriate care.

Normally when we wish to achieve a certain objective we establish criteria to help us in making the specific judgments necessary to achieve that objective. For example, if the objective of the NHS is to maximise health gain, then a criterion including quality adjusted life years might be appropriate. However, given that the objectives of the NHS are multiple and likely to be conflicting it is difficult to establish which criteria are relevant for each objective or group of objectives. Furthermore, when we consider the public benefits we may be unsure how precisely to achieve objectives related to these benefits.

Box 2: Personal benefits in full

Mortality related

- Lives saved (for example, in preventive medicine)
- Survival beyond some specified life stage (for example, intensive care unit deaths, hospital deaths, perioperative deaths, infant mortality, deaths in childbirth)
- Survival beyond some specified time point (for example, one year survival rates)
- Improved life expectancy (for example, life years gained)

Morbidity related

Presence or absence of:

- Disease (for example, prevalence or incidence of stroke, breast cancer, etc)
- Abnormal state (for example, organ or system dysfunction)
- Symptom (for example, dizziness, nausea, pain, rash)
- Psychological abnormality

Health related quality of life

Reduction of or adaption to:

- Abnormal feelings (for example, dizziness, nausea, pain, depression, anxiety)
- Restricted physical capacity (for example, mobility, lifting, self care)
- Restricted sensory capacity (for example, sight, hearing, touch, smell)
- Restricted mental capacity (for example, speech, understanding, memory)
- Restricted social capacity (activities of daily living, work, leisure activities)

Composites (usually combining mortality with one of the others)

- Symptom free life expectancy
- Healthy active life expectancy
- Disability adjusted life years
- Quality adjusted life years

Satisfaction

- With structure (for example, with facilities provided)
- With process (for example, with time spent waiting in the outpatient department, fairness of the decision making process, courtesy, information)
- With outcome (defined in one or other of the ways listed above)

Morally related benefits

There are also "morally related" benefits that need to be taken into account, such as respect for individual autonomy and respect for individual equal moral worth. These could be located within "satisfaction with process" but are emphasised separately because of their importance

It is, however, possible to outline criteria—all based in some way on characteristics of people (including the effects of healthcare interventions on them)—which are generally considered to be candidates for discriminating between competing claims for resources. These relate to questions of how to allocate the personal benefits outlined above. The NHS can concentrate on improving the health of the following possible groups:

- The whole population as much as possible (based on cost effectiveness measures)

- People most in need—those with the greatest illness or ill health deficit (for example, triage)
- Particular disadvantaged groups (for example, ethnic minority communities)
- People on whom others depend (for example, those with dependent children)
- People whose contribution to society is highly valued (for example, an eminent scientist)
- People who "deserve" it (for example, those who avoid unhealthy lifestyles)
- People who have been waiting the longest
- Particular age groups (for example, people who have most of their lives still before them).

Which of these criteria (and the objectives with which they are associated) are ethically defensible and which are not? Can we assign weights to those that are defensible? Whatever the answers there will always be a need to be sensitive to costs—that is, every choice to treat one person involves a loss of the benefits available to others. Cost is therefore an underlying constraint on all the objectives of the NHS.

There are two final questions in relation to ethics. The first concerns justice to providers: how much can we expect from those who provide healthcare in the context of implementing rationing decisions? Fair treatment of providers may be a proper constraint on what can and should be done to ration healthcare. Second, what proportion of current resources should be allocated to future benefits? In other words, what priority should we give to innovative treatments and to research?

Case study: Jaymee Bowen ("Child B")

Jaymee Bowen, aged 10 ("Child B" at the centre of the recent legal controversy) had acute myeloid leukaemia. She was given some initial treatment, including a bone marrow transplant at the Royal Marsden Hospital, but after a remission her cancer recurred. NHS clinicians at Addenbrooke's Hospital, Cambridge, decided that further bone marrow transplantation was inappropriate—that the probability of a successful outcome was very slight (2·5%) and that treatment would cause considerable pain and distress. However, on advice from abroad that further treatment and a second transplant still offered a significant chance of success Jaymee's father pressed for another transplant, this time from the Hammersmith Hospital, London. Cambridge Health Authority refused to pay for the extracontractual referral that this entailed on the basis that clinicians at both Addenbrooke's and the Hammersmith thought the treatment was unlikely to succeed and would cause considerable pain and distress.

Jaymee's father took the case to the high court, where Mr Justice Laws required the health authority to reconsider. However, on appeal the health authority's decision was upheld. Cambridge Health Authority consistently argued that financial matters did not enter its decision. Treatment was finally offered in the private sector, by Dr P J Gravett at the London Clinic, but again Cambridge Health Authority declined to pay.[4]

The case provoked considerable public attention, including several offers to pay for the treatment, one of which was accepted. However, the treatment ultimately provided by Dr Gravett was not bone marrow transplantation but a leading edge treatment—namely, donor lymphocyte infusion. Only about 20 patients have received this treatment and Jaymee is thought to have been the only child. The treatment sets up a graft versus host reaction which is intended to attack the cancer cells. It also attacks other parts of the body, such as cells within the lungs. The treatment was effective for a while and the cancer went into remission for over a year. It eventually recurred, however, and in May 1996 Jaymee died.

Several issues in this case relate to our agenda, but first we must distinguish one that does not. Imagine the proposed treatment for Jaymee had cost only one penny: would it still be in her interest? If there is a very low probability of benefit associated with a definite possibility of harm it may not be appropriate to offer treatment—or it might, in any event, be refused by the patient. Establishing the facts relating to the probability of benefit from a treatment and who should be included in making the decision on whether certain risks should be borne—the child, her parents, the doctors, the health authority—are important issues, but they are not questions about rationing. The health authority claimed that it had declined to fund further treatment solely on these grounds even though the family and child concerned desired it.

However, the proposed treatments did cost a substantial sum—for example, £75 000 for the second bone marrow transplantation. Regardless of the health authority's insistence that its decision was made only on grounds of appropriateness, there is nevertheless a rationing issue about whether it is ethically defensible to use resources in cases with very small probabilities of success and significant probabilities of harm: could more good be done elsewhere? Or is the degree of ill health or "need" in an individual case an important enough criterion to weigh against the good forgone to others? Does refusing to finance treatment in individual cases such as this damage the benefit of reassurance which the NHS provides? Are these sorts of judgments applied consistently across the NHS and is there sufficient explicitness to judge?

Furthermore, should special consideration be given to treatments that are innovative and promise tangible future benefits? There may be a case for setting aside a special budget for very leading edge treatments when there is a difficult balance of harm and benefit. The treatment which Jaymee Bowen eventually received is not the most expensive in the NHS, and without experiment knowledge will not advance. On the other hand, the prognosis in Jaymee's case was not good. Her life was extended by little over a year and she suffered considerable distress towards the end. Who should decide whether funds should be allocated to these experimental treatments?

Democracy

Ethical debates are extremely unlikely to result in unanimity. Though rational discussion is possible, personal values and innate feelings will often prove resistant to change and may remain persistently polarised among members of a society. In this context there is a need to develop democratic systems of decision making in order to resolve conflicts. The issues of democracy relate to how rationing should be conducted so as to conform to prevailing notions of democratic accountability.

Whose values might be taken into account?

Given that values are likely to vary widely among members of a society, whose values might be taken into account? Box 1 gives the list of possible candidates. It would probably be difficult to defend a position which gave absolutely no weight to the views of a particular section of the population. Hence the question becomes one of deciding on the appropriate weighting and combination of values rather than selecting which groups are relevant. We outline below some of the issues with various candidates.

17

The general public is a complex group. Incorporating the views of the general public will involve difficulties in establishing the appropriate perspective the people are to take—are they to speak, for example, as citizens, as potential patients, or as taxpayers?

Patients' values are clearly important in understanding how various medical interventions are valued by those receiving them. Patients may, however, be biased towards their own needs in deciding between rival claims.

Patients' families and friends may articulate excessive demands for overly aggressive treatment. On the other hand, they are best placed to articulate the values and needs of those close to them who cannot speak for themselves.

Interest and user groups may tend to speak for the most articulate or overrepresent the views of patients with fairly common diseases. However, they are often best placed to articulate the values of their constituencies.

Clinicians may value treatments because they are part of their professional work but which are nevertheless of no benefit or may actually be harmful.

Managers' values will inevitably feed into the decision making process and like other professionals managers may hide decisions from the public. However, both clinicians and managers are well placed to understand the nature of the choices which need to be made.

Central government politicians must have an input as they are elected to implement policies related to a (broad) set of values. However, they may wish to avoid certain difficult issues, and governments of any complexion may be too prone to short term expediency for their values to reflect the long term interests of citizens.

Local government representatives do not currently have a means for directly communicating their values. Ought they to have more influence in order to reflect the views of their community or would this cause an unhelpful conflict with central politicians' values? Are they also subject to the same concerns as those mentioned above in relation to central government?

"Experts" should inform the debate rather than promote their own values. But might we give special weight to those who are dedicated to studying questions of value judgment—ethicists, for example?

18

Media The values of the media will inevitably shape the context in which the rationing debate takes place. Though the media are well placed to communicate the values of otherwise marginalised groups or individuals, they will also be motivated by concerns relating to audience satisfaction, which may be less appropriate to rationing issues.

Industry's values need to be understood as they will inevitably have a strong influence—for example, through advertising strategies. Industry, however, will be motivated in large measure by commercial imperatives, which are not relevant to rationing in the NHS.

Groups with "moral authority" such as the clergy, could have their values given undue weight simply because of their position. However, they may have a role in speaking for the otherwise inarticulate disadvantaged.

The judiciary can play a part in distilling principles from test cases, thus providing an opportunity for others to endorse or reject such interpretations.

Who should have responsibility for making rationing decisions?

If the appropriate weighting of values of all the various groups can be established they will then need to be implemented. In other words, someone will always need to actually make the hard choices in allocating resources. But rationing decisions can be made in many different contexts and at many different levels within the NHS. Furthermore, in each of these contexts and at each of these levels certain groups listed in Box 1 could be given more or less responsibility for making choices. There is therefore clearly a normative question relating to who should have responsibility for making rationing decisions and in which situations.

Taking the range of possible groups listed in Box 1 as our starting point, we outline below the issues for some of these groups.

The general public might not be appropriate to actually make decisions (as opposed to provide a value input) owing to problems of establishing representativeness. They may also lack adequate expertise in matters of technical complexity. However, citizens' juries and other participatory devices offer a mechanism for including "lay" judgment more directly into rationing decisions.

Healthcare professionals have traditionally (and implicitly) undertaken the bulk of rationing decisions in the NHS, particularly on day to day matters.

The NHS reforms have weakened this influence. Is it still too strong, guided by vested interests? Or would further weakening adversely affect the ability of clinicians to make appropriate decisions in individual cases?

Managers traditionally have had comparatively little influence in rationing matters, though with the development of the purchasing function in the NHS this has changed somewhat. Should they have more—for example, by promoting clinical guidelines with a managerial perspective? Or does this intrude on the proper role of the clinician?

Central government makes decisions on how finance is distributed around Britain and sets the legal context. Should it do more and develop a national framework for rationing? Or is this inappropriate and should the NHS operate in a more locally driven way?

Local government representatives may arguably be a more appropriate group for making rationing decisions given their elected status and responsibility for other care agencies. However, this might cause difficulties for a national health strategy, geographical equity, and allocating finance between "free" healthcare and means tested social care.

"Experts" and groups with "moral authority" might be given a greater role in advising on clear, rational, and morally informed decision making at all levels. On the other hand, this might give too much influence to a particular set of interests.

The judiciary will inevitably make decisions when a point of law is in dispute. Should this role be encouraged as a check on the actions of other groups? Or is it important that the courts should be used only as a last resort?

What accountability mechanisms are appropriate?

Once the appropriate allocation of responsibilities for implementing rationing decisions has been established it will be necessary to institute appropriate mechanisms for ensuring that these decisions are made in a proper manner. This is the role of accountability mechanisms. Accountability entails both giving an account of the decisions that have been or are planned to be taken, and the operation or threat of sanctions so that those making decisions can be properly controlled.

Accountability mechanisms can be organised into four separate categories—political, organisational, public pressure, and normative.[1]

Political methods are the most formal and are based on the authority of the sovereign lawmaking body—parliament and European lawmaking bodies. They include agencies and strategies at the disposal of (1) the legislature (for example, review of funding, review of statutory instruments, Health Select Committee, Health Service Commissioner, National Audit Office); (2) the political executive (for example, fiscal powers, Social Services Inspectorate, Health Advisory Service, Audit Commission, personnel appointments, 1991 reforms); and (3) the judiciary (for example, Mental Health Review Tribunal, judicial review).

Organisational methods entail the NHS regulating itself, either by strengthening internal discipline and good management (for example, the development of general management within the NHS), or by exercising "open" government and exposing itself to the influence of publicity and the scrutiny of the media (for example, by publishing how health authority decisions were made or instituting a citizens' jury), or through the operation of a quasimarket system.

Public pressure mechanisms include the activity of pressure groups and complaints mechanisms (for example, SANE, Patients Association, NHS complaints procedure) and statutory bodies (for example, community health councils) as well as the possibility of individual patients switching from one agency to another (for example, changing doctor).

Normative methods include the inculcation of public service ethos within individuals or professional groups, who then police themselves according to internal codes of conduct (clinicians' ethical codes and peer sanction). Systems of clinical audit might also be implemented to promote normative accountability.

In the past the political methods have been the most influential. One option for improving accountability is to continue to develop these political instruments by giving more power to watchdogs such as the Audit Commission or the select committee. Alternatively, more radical methods could be introduced. More of the decision making process could be undertaken in public and the reasons for decisions published more extensively. Aided by the media, this would allow more public scrutiny—though increased openness might make decision making more difficult and encourage "capture" by pressure groups. Citizens' juries offer another mechanism for giving the public more influence over the decision making process. But this could encourage the statutory decision making authority to evade its legal responsibility as the final arbiter and thereby weaken accountability. Another option might be for the purchasing role in the NHS to be given over to elected local authorities. But this may, for example, make it more difficult to develop an integrated "national" health policy. Finally, accountability might be improved by exploiting the potential for clinical audit to ensure that clinical decisions are consistent with NHS policies. However, this would require the results of clinical audit to be made available to managers; some doctors may consider that these matters should be kept within the peer review network.

Clearly, accountability requires adequate information. This issue is revisited below.

How explicit should be the principles by which rationing is conducted?

We established at the beginning of this paper that one of our substantive positions is that the principles by which rationing decisions are taken should be more explicit. One mechanism for improving accountability mentioned above—that of openness—would automatically encourage a more explicit debate, which we support. However, there are important issues relating to the degree to which explicitness and openness are necessarily helpful, particularly for the working of the NHS.

Those who argue for retaining a degree of implicitness cite the following:

- Rationing is morally and methodologically impossible to resolve to everyone's satisfaction. The trust the public currently has in the medical profession could be damaged by the explicit acknowledgment of this. Furthermore, the public could make matters worse by becoming directly involved
- Such a situation could threaten public confidence in the NHS, particularly if individual cases or forms of treatment were excluded publicly on the basis of "abstract" principles
- Being explicit about principles cannot accommodate the heterogeneous nature of healthcare and the complexity of individual cases.

On the other hand, those who favour explicitness argue that:

- In a democracy citizens must be allowed to influence decision making, both to develop their own moral commitment to democracy and in order to improve decision making itself by providing feedback to decision makers
- By being explicit vested interests are discouraged from making decisions on the basis of tradition, prejudice, or whim or in response to vocal, articulate, powerful, or wealthy groups

- If rationing is "messy", then it is better to be open about this than to risk the consequences of deceiving the public
- Explicit principles do not codify behaviour, they merely place moral boundaries on the decisions to be taken in individual cases.

Case study: Treatment of an elderly dying woman

An 81 year old woman was admitted to a short stay geriatric ward confused and ill after falling at home. During her stay she developed diarrhoea and oral thrush. Staff were under pressure and unable to care adequately for these conditions; at one point the woman was claimed to have been handled roughly. It became clear the woman was dying, and the lack of privacy was distressing for both patient and family. The hospital looked decayed and dirty.

In a case like this it can be difficult to disentangle incompetence and improper behaviour from issues of rationing. No patient should ever be handled roughly. However, the context of these events is determined by rationing decisions elsewhere in the system. In particular, what weight should be given to allocating resources for the care of elderly patients? It may be that resources should be devoted to young people as they have greater life expectancy. Or should age play no part in these decisions? And within the budget assigned to the care of elderly patients is enough weight given to dignity and respect for autonomy—or should resources be devoted to improving symptoms or life expectancy?

Such decisions are often highly implicit—that is, it is not clear who is responsible or why decisions have been taken—with consequent implications for accountability. This raises questions about whose values should count in allocating resources between client groups: why does geriatrics seem to have a low priority? Is it because of public and professional pressure to supply resources to more glamorous areas of medicine?

We have stated our position in favour of being open and explicit in terms of rationing issues. Whatever principles are thought to be appropriate should be articulated publicly, and these should constitute the framework within which rationing takes place—though the Rationing Agenda Group does not collectively hold a view about what these principles should be.

Nevertheless, there remain important issues around the degree of explicitness in specifying principles that is sensible or possible and the degree to which these principles should be articulated in the context of an individual consultation.

Empirical issues

Empirical or factual issues include fairly uncontroversial questions relating to descriptive analyses of how the process of rationing currently

Case study: Interferon-β

Interferon-β is a drug for the relapsing–remitting form of multiple sclerosis. Evidence for licensing the drug comes from a single trial which showed that it seemed to reduce the number of exacerbations of the disease by about one third but had no effect on progression. There have been doubts about the methodology used in the trial. The drug is expected to cost about £10 000 per patient a year. There are estimated to be 85 000 patients with multiple sclerosis in the UK. Of these, 45% are thought to have the relapsing–remitting form. If all these patients were treated the total cost could be £380m—that is, 10% of the drug bill.[5]

Evidence for the efficacy of interferon-β is weak and disputed. More information is necessary about its costs and benefits in order to hold those who make decisions on its use accountable. Licensing authorities do not need to take account of evidence on cost effectiveness when granting a licence.

Even given the best evidence available, is expenditure on interferon-β a good use of NHS resources? It seems likely that more benefit could be derived elsewhere from the resources required; however, a specific group would be denied potentially beneficial treatment. If some health authorities declined to fund it what implications would this have for the NHS objective of geographical equity? How should the values of those authorities be weighed against the values of others in assessing the resources to be devoted to this drug? A key question is who should be responsible for undertaking rationing. Once licensed, a drug can in general be prescribed by any doctor. If this is a general practitioner the budget will not be cash limited and resources may be taken from other areas of the NHS without the general practitioner taking this into account. On the other hand, hospital neurologists operate under cash limits. Should clinicians' freedom to prescribe be further limited by the health authority? Should the government have a role? (An executive letter was circulated to health authorities advising on the introduction of interferon-β.) What role should the judiciary have? It may have a role in adjudicating if an individual doctor prescribes against the advice of the health authority or central government.

Accountability mechanisms seem weak. The work of the licensing authority is not widely publicised. If individual clinicians take the rationing decisions there are few mechanisms for ensuring the proper democratic control of their actions. If the health authority attempts to restrain prescribing its legal position is unclear. Health authority decisions may not themselves be made in an accountable manner.

Finally, many decisions related to the rationing of interferon-β are likely to be made in a highly secretive way. Improved information is needed in order to make the process more explicit and accountable. But what implications are there for being explicit in individual consultations if only a few courses of the drug are available for prescription in any one location? Will this damage trust in the doctor–patient relationship or encourage a mature and responsible partnership?

works in practice in the NHS. But they also include issues relating to how much information is necessary to make rationing more accountable and whether we have enough knowledge to implement specific rationing strategies.

Who undertakes rationing and what mechanisms are used?

Any group listed in Box 1 might influence rationing decisions because their values are taken into account directly, because they constitute part of an accountability mechanism, or because they influence the system in some other way. But in practice the bulk of rationing decisions in the NHS as it currently operates are taken by either clinicians or managers. In addition, central government sets the overall framework for making choices by specifying how purchasing power is distributed to regions. Central government also issues annual planning and priorities guidelines, executive letters, and exhortatory initiatives (such as those relating to waiting lists) and sets the legal framework for charging and the overall range of NHS responsibilities.

If rationing is taking place those concerned must be making use of mechanisms, whether formal or informal, statutorily based, or administrative. The following suggestions about how rationing is effected in practice are split among the national, institutional, and individual levels.

At the *national level* rationing is effected by (1) changes to the legal framework (for example, allocating tax revenue between NHS and other health promoting activities, such as housing policy); (2) exercising executive powers (for example, devising geographical allocation formulae and setting prescription charges); and (3) specific initiatives (for example, *Health of the Nation* and the annual planning and priorities guidance).

At the *institutional level* rationing is effected by (1) government agencies exercising delegated authority in allocating resources—for example, health authorities commissioning care (and possibly excluding services such as cosmetic surgery) and making decisions on extracontractual referrals; (2) pricing (for example, of packages of care to be purchased by health authorities; and (3) managed care strategies (for example, clinical guidelines).

At the *individual level* the general practitioner acts as the principal "gatekeeper" to care in the NHS. This serves to mediate the delivery of care both between doctor and patient and between generalist and specialist clinicians. But whenever an individual patient comes into contact with the NHS one of five methods may be used to bring the demand for care into line with the available supply[2]—namely:

- Denial—that is, not providing treatment at all for more or less justifiable reasons (for example, refusal by certain general practitioners to register homeless people or drug abusers and non-provision of treatments claimed to be ineffective or inappropriate)
- Deflection—that is, encouragement to use other agencies for care (for example, substitution of "social" care for "health" care for patients with long term needs)
- Delay—that is, not providing all forms of care immediately, which provides a kind of holding area to "buffer" excess demand (for example, waiting to obtain a general practitioner or consultant appointment; waiting lists for secondary care; and waiting in accident and emergency departments)
- Dilution—that is, reducing quality in order that existing resources may go further; this may or may not also represent a more efficient use of resources (for example, by not using the most expensive prostheses or downgrading the skillmix in nursing teams)
- Deterrence—even when services are nominally "free" there will be certain costs to individual patients which may deter them from seeking care (for example, distance, such as living a long way from a general practitioner's premises; poor information or information only in English; and hostile staff or environments).

Among other mechanisms, a lottery system could be implemented in certain circumstances to make a choice between claims considered to be morally equal; and a system of rights could be instituted whereby choices would need to be made with reference to a codified system of individual entitlements to healthcare adjudicated by the judicial system.[3]

What additional information would be required to make rationing more explicit and those responsible more accountable? Is there sufficient knowledge to implement particular rationing strategies successfully?

There is little doubt that more information and knowledge would help rationing. It is also clear that rationing needs to take place whatever the quality of the information available—there is no question of there being insufficient information to ration. Information can never be complete and we will always be operating with a less than perfect understanding of the state of the world. Indeed, striving for perfect information may not itself be a sensible goal: collecting information entails costs, which means that resources cannot be used to provide benefits of other kinds.

The first question posed above therefore relates to this last point: where should there be a priority for improving the level of information in order to improve explicit and accountable rationing? Possible aspects in which improved information might be valuable include the following:

- Population health status—that is, the current distribution of disease, disability, illness, and risk factors
- Healthcare requirements—that is, those needs that are amenable to healthcare interventions

Case study: In vitro fertilisation

In a study of 114 purchasing plans for 1992–3, six health authorities explicitly stated that they would not be buying in vitro fertilisation or gamete intrafallopian transfer (GIFT) treatment for their populations. At the same time other purchasers were continuing to buy in vitro fertilisation and some even planned to put extra money into the service.[6] For some purchasing authorities this issue was one of relevance—is in vitro fertilisation the sort of intervention (does it produce the sort of benefit) that is relevant to the business of the NHS? Arguably, inability to conceive is not an illness and if people wish to benefit from in vitro fertilisation they should purchase it in the private sector. On the other hand, there is clearly some physiological dysfunction and there may be severe psychological distress. Does this not indicate a medical condition for which the NHS should take responsibility?

If in vitro fertilisation is considered relevant to the NHS, then the question of allocating resources arises. In particular, does geographical equity demand that all health authorities should provide some level of service so that a patient's place of residence does not have a decisive influence on the likelihood of treatment? How should the benefits of in vitro fertilisation be weighed against those of other treatments if some level of provision is required? In this context who should make choices about its provision? If health authorities and clinicians are responsible for providing the service some localities may have no service at all; if the government institutes a national policy this will dilute the local nature of decision making in the NHS.

Whose values should count in whether or not to include in vitro fertilisation as an NHS service? Certain sections of the population may not be sympathetic—for example, men and people who do not desire children. Furthermore, some doctors may not view infertility as an illness. On the other hand, those patients unable to conceive and their friends and representatives may value their own needs highly simply because they have direct experience of the condition.

Though only a few health authorities have explicitly stated they will not purchase fertility services, there may be others that are doing so implicitly. Is this an appropriate way for decisions to be taken in the NHS? What sort of information and how much more do we require for these decisions to be more open? How can accountability be exercised in this setting?

- Degree of need or ill health deficit—that is, information about relative degrees of need in different groups
- Capacity to benefit—that is, information about the relative effectiveness of various interventions (for example, information relating to individual preferences or utilities for health states as one measure of benefit)
- Cost—that is, information about the costs of various interventions
- Current provision—that is, information about what is currently provided and why, as a basis for making appropriate changes in the future.

There may also be a need to improve the level of information about how rationing is conducted now: what principles and criteria are currently being used to make choices? Furthermore, there is the question of how much effort should be devoted to attempting to elicit, through various research methods, an accurate understanding of what people's values actually are.

This leads to the second question: do we have enough information or knowledge to undertake certain strategies with reference to rationing? For a strategy to succeed there needs to be clarity about the objective. As we have seen, there is little consensus about what the objectives of the NHS are. And attempts to collect some kinds of information may be so beset with difficulties that we should proceed with caution in using them for rationing decisions to ensure that they do not lead to worse outcomes than by simply continuing with more familiar data.

Incrementalist models of decision making argue that "synoptic" decision making, which strives for completeness, may end with worse outcomes than by "muddling through". However, there is clearly a need to improve the levels of information and knowledge at our disposal to improve explicitness and accountability. We must ensure that the best available data are deployed even if they are imperfect, for everything else is bound to be worse. The appropriate balance needs to be struck.

How does the system of financing healthcare affect the practice of rationing?

One response to the proposition at the beginning of this chapter—that rationing is inevitable—is to argue that if we altered the system of financing then we might avoid the problem of rationing altogether. This kind of argument assumes that rationing occurs only in cash limited, taxation based systems such as the NHS. In fact, all healthcare systems entail allocating scarce resources among those who might benefit; all include rationing in this sense.

Private insurance based systems ration care by making households decide how much of their resources they wish to spend on premiums; some may wish to spend none. Tax based systems which introduce charges also partly shift the burden of payment out of government budgets directly on to households; "earmarked" contributions are forms of disguised taxation. But all involve decisions about how to use households' resources.

The only difference will be in the particular set of financial incentives that affect the people concerned. In a largely private, insurance based system such as that in the USA this may encourage inefficiency—that is, oversupply for some and no supply for others. Social insurance systems such as those in France and Germany may also be overresourced. Proposing other forms of finance is no escape from the fundamental issue. It merely alters the way in which the people concerned respond to inevitable scarcity.

In conclusion it is worth making clear that we do not propose any fundamental changes in the methods by which the NHS is financed. We support the continuation of a publicly financed NHS. However, we wish to promote an ongoing, open, and informed debate on how to make the hard choices about who should benefit from its limited resources.

The original signatories to this document were: Dr Robert Maxwell (Chair), King's Fund, London; Mr John Cairns, University of Aberdeen; Dr Nan Carle, King's Fund Management College, London; Dr Angela Coulter, King's Fund Development Centre, London; Professor Len Doyal, St Bartholomew's and the London Hospital School of Medicine and Dentistry, London; Professor John Gabbay, University of Southampton; Professor Raanan Gillon, Imperial College, London; Ms Heather Goodare, Horsham; Dr Iona Heath, Kentish Town Health Centre, London; Mr Chris Heginbotham, East and North Hertfordshire Health Authority, Welwyn Garden City; Mr John James, Kensington and Chelsea and Westminister Health Commissioning Agency, London; Professor Alison Kitson, Royal College of Nursing, London; Professor Alan Maynard, University of York; Professor Sheila McLean, University of Glasgow; Rabbi Julia Neuberger, London; Mr Bill New, King's Fund Policy Institute, London; Ms Marianne Rigge, College of Health, London; Mr Nick Ross, London; Professor Peter Rubin, Queen's Medical Centre, Nottingham; Dr Richard Smith, *BMJ*, London; Professor Albert Weale, University of Essex; Professor Alan Williams, University of York; Ms Karen Brown, London.

1 Peters BG. *The politics of bureaucracy*. 3rd edn London: Longman, 1989.
2 Harrison S, Hunter D. *Rationing health care*. London: Institute for Public Policy Research, 1994.

3 Doyal L. Needs, rights and equity: moral quality in healthcare rationing. *Quality in Health Care* 1995;4:273–83.
4 Maxwell R, ed. *Rationing health care*. London: Churchill Livingstone, 1995.
5 Walley T, Barton S. A purchaser perspective of managing new drugs: interferon beta as a case study. *BMJ* 1995;311:796–9.
6 Redmayne S, Klein R. Rationing in practice: the case of in vitro fertilisation. *BMJ* 1993; 306:1521–4.

3 Responses to *The Rationing Agenda in the NHS*

JO LENAGHAN

General

The Rationing Agenda Group (RAG) was founded to deepen the debate on rationing health care. To this end, a short document was produced in 1996 in an attempt to set out as neutrally as possible all the issues that the group felt should be considered when debating the rationing of health care.[1] The RAG document was published as an article in the *BMJ* and circulated to all stakeholders, who were invited to forward any comments or suggestions to the authors. The RAG received a wide range of correspondence from clinicians, health authorities, Community Health Councils (CHCs), health economists, industry, and politicians, as well as interested observers and practitioners from abroad. A total of 82 letters was received, and the following chapter is an attempt to give a flavour of the kind of responses that the RAG document provoked and to identify key areas of consensus and difference for further debate.

Most responses to the objectives of RAG in general and the document in particular were overwhelmingly positive. Many respondents shared the sentiments of Dr Gillian Ford, Medical Director of Marie Curie Cancer Care, who welcomed the document as

> A very clear and well set out summary which can well serve as an agenda for the discussion. It is crisp and stimulating and recognises the difference between setting a framework for a difficult discussion and trying to settle the issues.

Mr John Hudson, Dean of the School for Health Care Studies, Leeds, praised the document as a major contribution to the debate on rationing of health care provision:

31

It is an important first step which has already moved RAG towards its aim of raising the quality of debate on the issue.

The framework of analysis offered by RAG, although welcomed by the majority, was felt to be less than helpful by some. Philip Rhodes (retired, Professor of Gynaecology, St Thomas' Hospital) argued that

> Clinicians feel assailed on all sides by the sorts of people on (the) Rationing Agenda Group who have no direct experience of the clinical situations, but who are constantly ready with advice and criticism.

However, several clinicians and managers wrote to confirm that the issues outlined in the article confronted them every day in their work and seemed to welcome the attention that RAG gave these dilemmas. Dr CM Tomkins, Professional Services Director of the MDU, explained:

> We are often contacted by our members for advice about situations in which issues of rationing in health care arise... These situations do cause clinicians real difficulties and we hope this area will receive attention and debate...

Overall, most respondents welcomed the RAG publication, as well as the aims and objectives of the Group in furthering the debate about rationing. There was a surprising degree of support for the two substantive positions taken by RAG, first that rationing is inevitable and second that the public should be made aware of this and have their views heard in the debate. As is evident from what follows, however, this apparent consensus begins to fracture once more detailed issues are addressed, such as what do we mean by rationing, what criteria should be used, to what extent should the public be involved and to what end?

Is rationing inevitable?

The Rationing Agenda Group deliberately chose to use the word "rationing" as a summary term "because it provokes the greatest public controversy". Surprisingly, not a single respondent objected to the terminology or argued for the more user friendly term "priority setting" so favoured by politicians. Janet Nash was the only correspondent to draw attention to this issue, arguing:

> I feel that the distinction between rationing and priority setting is difficult to make and is more to do with rationing having a base line. Procedures below that line are not available ... priority setting in the context of rationing means that procedures low on the list may or may not be funded, according to the availability of money.

The first substantive position taken by RAG was that the rationing of health care is inevitable. The overwhelming majority of respondents, including clinicians, managers, CHCs, church leaders, and MPs, agreed that this was the case and that, indeed, health care has always been rationed in the NHS. Ann Windiate, Chief Executive of the Riverside Mental Health Trust, wrote

I am convinced, having come to the NHS from 25 years in local authority social services, that rationing of health care is not only inevitable but has in fact been traditionally performed.

Many clinicians sent in case studies from their own practice as examples of the rationing dilemmas that they have to face every day. MJ Lowe, Deputy Secretary of the BMA, explained that

The BMA already has a policy on rationing which calls for an acceptance of rationing as inevitable.

He also argued that "rationing" should be defined more narrowly than the RAG proposed, in order for a meaningful debate to take place on the fundamental issues it raises.* Politicians are often accused of trying to duck the difficult issues associated with rationing, but Marion Roe, MP, Chairman of the House of Commons Select Committee on Health, wrote to point our that

... we also recognised that the need to set priorities in the NHS has been, and always will be with us.[2]

Although most respondents agreed that rationing has always been a feature of the NHS, some felt that there are certain features that distinguish rationing in the 1990s from that which has occurred in the past. Dr John Wilkinson, Consultant Dermatologist and Medical Director at South Bucks NHS Trust, claimed that historically rationing was mainly "medical" in nature with decisions made on the basis of a clinical assessment of co-morbidity, age/life expectancy, quality of life, etc.

Today, he claimed, clinicians are having to ration on a purely "budgetary" basis. Others, such as Ross Tristem, Director of the NHS Trust Federation, suggested that rationing is becoming an increasingly urgent issue in the 1990s as a result of policies such as the waiting list initiative and the Patients' Charter, which have helped to fuel patient expectations.

---

* The BMA suggested the following definition: Rationing involves the denial of treatment on grounds other than simple clinical judgment. The treatment being denied is assumed to otherwise improve the individual's quality of life. Therefore, denial of treatment on grounds of clinical judgment is not rationing, and denial of treatment which would have no beneficial effect is not rationing. Rationing then becomes an issue of affordability versus treatments which are to varying extents beneficial.

Not all correspondents, however, agreed with the RAG's substantive view that rationing is inevitable. Some argued that, instead of looking at how to ration, we should first of all examine whether we need to ration at all. Colin Roberts, Professor of Epidemiology and Public Health, University of Wales College of Medicine, wrote to explain the work of the Anti-Rationing Group (ARG) which consists of people from all parts of the NHS who share the belief that the rationing of effective health care is unnecessary and that, if it is allowed to occur, will lead to the destruction of the NHS.[3] He argued that denying treatment known to be effective, while at the same time allowing present levels of over-buying, blind buying and over-pricing to go unchallenged, is unacceptable, if not immoral. Several people, such as Neil Doverty, NHS Management Trainee at Kingston Hospital, although mainly agreeing with the RAG's substantive view on rationing, suggested that the RAG should in future address the issues raised by the ARG with as much fervour as they state the inevitability of rationing. Although the objective of the RAG is explicitly to argue that rationing is inevitable, a substantial minority of respondents felt that the RAG would have more credibility and influence if they addressed the arguments of their opponents in greater detail.

Some respondents questioned whether the need to ration would be removed if the NHS funding mechanism was changed or the level of resources increased. The RAG acknowledged that an increase in funding would undoubtedly result in a different threshold at which rationing occurred, but claimed that hard choices would still have to be made and that the same fundamental issues would still be at stake. Is it enough to insist that "rationing is inevitable"? Are certain kinds or degrees of rationing more inevitable and more or less acceptable than others? Is Kate Mackay, Consultant in Public Health Medicine, right to highlight the difference between having to wait for 4–6 months for a hernia repair and waiting 12–24 months? The letters both in support of and against the inevitability of rationing revealed the complexity of issues that lie behind this apparently simple substantive position and point to the need for further exploration of these issues.

Should rationing be explicit?

Of the majority that agreed with the substantive position that rationing is inevitable, the question of whether or not the principles upon which rationing decisions are based should be made explicit provoked a lively response. Most appeared to agree with the RAG's second substantive position that whatever principles are thought to be appropriate should be articulated publicly and the views of the public should be heard in the debate. Some, such as Colin Roberts, felt that the public should be "educated about how rationing could be avoided and made aware of the likely consequences if it is not." Others, such as Jane Western, Chair of East Wiltshire Health Care, felt that the public voice should be "heard". Some respondents argued that the public should be involved in actual rationing decisions (see below).

There was much less agreement about whether the actual practice of rationing at the micro level should be made explicit: how and why it is done in all individual circumstances. The RAG itself did not take a view on the extent to which any principles should be articulated in the context of an individual consultation.

Some respondents argued that explicit rationing already exists. Dr Rhiannon Tudor Edwards, Lecturer in Health Economics, Department of Public Health, University of Liverpool, claimed that the move from implicit to explicit rationing is already under way in the management of elective waiting lists, giving immediacy to the philosophical and practical questions raised by the RAG.[4] Others, while supporting the objective of explicit rationing in principle, highlighted the difficulties of achieving this in practice. MJ Lowe, Deputy Secretary of the BMA, acknowledged that there is a case for making explicit those treatments that, although beneficial, will not be made available on cost grounds. He also argued, however, that the establishment of explicit criteria, no matter how well founded, will only delay the point at which clinical judgment comes into play and, as such judgment is always subject to uncertainty, it is probable that the exercise would fail, although he felt that this should not prevent us from discussing the issues.

Others questioned not just whether explicit rationing was possible, but whether it was indeed desirable. Professor Philip Rhodes wrote:

> My first inclination is to agree with the other proposition that "we need to be more explicit about the principles and issues" of rationing. Yet then I stopped to ask why? My question is intended to clarify rather than cloud the problem. Is it really a problem or is it best left alone as being virtually insoluble ...? Could it be that "muddling through" on the basis of individual decisions in various places where medicine is practised could be better in the long run than policies proposed from on high without full knowledge of individual circumstances? ... It may not be equitable, but must all patients everywhere have everything that everyone else does? Is life fair? Can it be made so?

There was little consensus around this issue in the letters sent to the RAG, and this again points to the need for further discussion and debate. At what level and to what extent (if any) should we be explicit about the principles by which rationing decisions are taken? More importantly, what is it that we hope to achieve? Do we expect explicit rationing to be more rational and/or more fair, or does this strategy represent an attempt to develop more legitimate, competent, and consensual decision making? If we argue against explicit rationing, are we trying to avoid or defuse potential conflicts and differences? Is it possible or desirable for rationing in practice, whether explicit or implicit, to be conflict free? These issues cut to the very heart of the rationing debate, which is perhaps why they are characterised by so much difference and division.

Involving the public

Richard Smith, Editor of the *BMJ*, pointed out in a letter to all the stakeholders:

> We have not gone as far as to say that the public should be involved in the rationing of health care, although I am sure that some members of RAG would adopt that position.

There were subtle but important differences of opinion among the respondents about the extent (if any) to which the public should be involved in rationing decisions and to what end. Some agreed with Ann Windiate, Chief Executive of the Riverside Mental Health Trust, that the public should be "consulted", whereas others, like Lyn Mitchell, Chief Executive of the National Board for Nursing, Midwifery and Health Visiting for Scotland, felt that the public should be "involved" in rationing decisions, or at least in developing the criteria upon which such judgments are made.

Although most respondents clearly supported some kind of public consultation in principle, several highlighted the practical difficulties of achieving this in practice. Jim Hill, Chairman of North Devon CHC, argued that

> It is difficult to involve the public, as people tend to focus on issues only when currently affected, whereas healthcare professionals are much better informed and are stimulated into thought/action on a daily basis . . . The trick seems to be to get the public, or a representative portion of it, to address these health issues in a sufficiently informed and structured way.

Dr Gillian Ford, Medical Director of Marie Curie Cancer Care, criticised the role of the media and the fact that public information seems to be confined to *causes célèbres* such as Jaymee Bowen (Child B) and the distorted public perceptions that this can result in.

The RAG acknowledged these problems and suggested that techniques such as citizens' juries may offer a way of involving the public in an informed way, but several correspondents expressed their scepticism about this method. Professor Philip Rhodes argued that

The concept of citizens' juries is just eyewash and sloppy thinking. There has been no clear thought given to their aims, objectives, remits and powers and methods of selection. The idea is just a sop to a vague idea of democracy.

Dr Roger Crisp, Fellow in Philosophy, St Anne's College, Oxford, questioned whether or not involving the public in rationing decisions would achieve the desired outcomes:

The rationale you give for democratic decision making is a good one—that it will decrease conflict. But encouraging a public debate may increase conflict, by politicising previously non-politicised issues.

This point was also made by Louise Locock, Research Associate at Templeton College, Oxford, who thought that public debate "wouldn't necessarily resolve conflicts any more effectively, even if it might be desirable for other reasons".

Clearly, there was a high degree of support for public involvement in principle, but perhaps more thought needs to be given to what we are trying to achieve by this strategy, and how it might best be achieved. Who are the public? Should they be educated, listened to, or involved in the decision making process itself? As Sir Douglas Black wrote, it is likely that all of these approaches may be appropriate to different kinds of rationing decisions at different kinds of levels. We need to develop a clear rationale for choosing between the options, rather than continuing to pay lip service to the need to involve the public in rationing debates and/or decisions.

Membership of the RAG

The RAG received several letters criticising or questioning the membership of the group. In particular, many people were critical of the apparent lack of practising medical professionals on the committee. RPH Thompson, Consultant Physician, wrote:

Searching through the signatories, I can find one GP and one Professor of Therapeutics. It seems strange that there is so little representation from clinicians as, after all, it is we who will have to face and discuss rationing with the patients, not health economists.

Professor Philip Rhodes shared this view, and a similar point was made by Jim Hill, Chairman of North Devon CHC, who wrote:

You will not be surprised if I note that the RAG has not availed itself of the experience of CHCs since they do not figure in the list of members of the group!

37

It is perhaps tempting to dismiss these complaints as those of the excluded. However, CJ Burns-Cox, Consultant Physician, Frenchay Healthcare Trust, Bristol, pointed out that clinicians and others would perhaps take a little more notice of the RAG

> if it included more people who actually had to face sick people and their families day by day over the years.

He also questioned the method of selection for members to sit in this group, arguing that its function should be more democratic.

It is hard to disagree with these points. If one of the purposes of the RAG is to provoke debate and build a consensus around issues concerned with rationing, then it must aim to build credibility not just through the quality of its work but by the selection and function of its committee.

Gaps in the agenda

The RAG was particularly keen for respondents to inform them of any issues that they felt should have been considered in the debate, but were overlooked. Several people responded to this request. MJ Lowe, Deputy Secretary of the BMA, expressed his surprise that

> the document makes no mention of the wider issues of public health policy that would prevent ill health and reduce the costs to the NHS. There needs to be consideration of the allocation of resources between areas such as education, transport, housing, etc. on a wider scale as they all have an impact on health.

This view was shared by Professor Trevor Sheldon, Director, NHS Centre for Reviews and Dissemination, University of York, who felt that it would have been useful if the RAG had referred in passing to rationing across, as well as between, areas of public expenditure:

> ... I am not sure of the legitimacy of even talking about healthcare rationing in isolation, if one of the aims is to maximise health gain and minimise health inequalities.

Professor Sheldon also felt that the RAG need to address the Anti-Rationing Group

> who think that rationing is purely a technical problem of eliminating waste. A strong paper on this is important. We must be careful that the legitimisation of rationing does not become a cover for those who will not address the issue of technical inefficiency ... take the 'rash' out of rationing!

He also argued that the RAG underestimated the implications of the system of financing for rationing.

> Different systems of financing may mobilise more (or fewer) resources and have an effect on the incidence of the burden and benefits ... this may require more study.

This view was also expressed by Professor Ray Robinson of Southampton University, who criticised the RAG for not considering the nature of rationing in a privately funded healthcare system. Indeed, although the RAG claimed to have only two substantive positions (that rationing is inevitable and the public should be involved in the debate), the document produced by the RAG also revealed a third substantive position—namely that the NHS should continue to be funded via general taxation.

Ralph Crawshaw, MD, Oregon, criticised the absence of any political analysis in the RAG document, arguing that "political receptor sites" need to be identified and the different power relationships analysed before even attempting to involve the public in a debate about rationing. Although this point was not raised by any other correspondent, it highlights an important gap that the RAG will have to fill if it intends to take the debate forward into the field of policy and action.

Furthering the debate

The RAG document succeeded in its attempt to further the debate about rationing, provoking 82 written responses from a wide range of stakeholders. Many bodies such as East Surrey Health Authority, East Wiltshire Health Care, the British Psychological Society, and the Free Church Federal Council used the document to facilitate debate within their own organisations. All correspondents expressed their support for the aims of the RAG in taking the debate forward. It is interesting to note that not one of the 82 letters received was from a member of the general public. This is perhaps not surprising, because of the forum in which the document was published and circulated. However, this raises important questions for the future. What mechanisms, channels, and language do we need to develop and exploit in order to encourage and facilitate such a debate? Indeed, do the public want to be involved?

There was a surprising degree of consensus among the respondents that rationing is inevitable, although a significant minority argued that if the RAG is to build credibility and a consensus for its views, it needs to respond to the arguments of the Anti-Rationing Group more rigorously, with particular reference to the consequences of altering the mechanism and/or level of funding. If the RAG is serious about involving the public in a debate about rationing, then this will be even more important. The public

39

will not be convinced if the RAG merely insists that rationing is inevitable—they will have to demonstrate that this has and always will be the case.

The apparent professional consensus about the inevitability of rationing did not survive the thornier questions of whether the principles upon which rationing decisions are based should be made explicit and, if so, to what degree and at what level. It would appear that, before we can decide how to ration (and therefore move into the realm of policy and action), we may need a more thorough debate about the purpose of the NHS and the appropriate balance between individual needs/demands and a collectively funded health service. These would seem appropriate issues for the public to start to enter into a debate and dialogue with professionals and patients. The work done by the RAG has provided a valuable opportunity for this process to begin.

1 New B, on behalf of the Rationing Agenda Group. The rationing agenda in the NHS. *BMJ* 1996;**312**:1593–601.
2 Roe, Marian. Politicians do not want to duch the issues. *BMJ* 1996;**313**:557.
3 Roberts, CJ. Anti-Rationing Group also want to contribute to the debate. *BMJ* 1996;**313**: 557.
4 Edwards, RT. Elective waiting lists are becoming explicitly rationed. *BMJ* 1996;**313**:558–9.

Section 1:
"Talk"

4 Why rationing is inevitable in the NHS

CHRIS HEGINBOTHAM

This chapter describes how rationing occurs currently in the National Health Service (NHS). There are those, notably the Anti-Rationing Group (ARG) and some health professionals, who believe that rationing would not be necessary if all procedures of unproven effectiveness were abandoned, and an emphasis was placed on evidence based medicine. These are laudable aims in themselves and will achieve improved efficiency and cost effectiveness of care. Unfortunately, rationing is so endemic within the NHS that these measures alone will be insufficient even with substantial investment in those areas where rationing is most obvious.

The contention here is that there will remain a need to ration healthcare for the foreseeable future, and this will not be affected more than marginally by any changes in the political complexion of national Government.[1] The boundaries of healthcare are so wide and elastic that there will always be a need to set priorities, however much money is pumped into the NHS. This chapter seeks to illustrate the extent of present rationing, and to demonstrate that simple mechanisms, although important and necessary in themselves, cannot remove the need for hard choices to be made.

There are many clear examples of rationing at present, some of which *would* disappear if sufficient resources were made available, although a lot would remain. Current rationing can be characterised in three main ways, set out in the box.

The first form of rationing is where there has historically been a simple underprovision of care, or where recent policy decisions have reduced the availability of straightforward diagnostic tests or effective treatments. Examples include dentistry and optometry. A related form of rationing is where constraints are placed on demand which will continue to grow if resources allow. For example, it is likely that people would use primary care services more if they were more readily available. Although this immediately raises questions about the effectiveness and appropriateness of particular forms of care, as expectations rise (fuelled, for instance, by

43

---

1 (a) Historic under-provision, or deliberate policy decisions to reduce availability of effective treatments free at point of delivery.

(b) Demand constraints on treatments of uncertain or unproven effectiveness but where patient expectations may be high.

2 Restrictions on leading edge, not fully tested but promising techniques or medicines, including experimental treatments.

3 Reduced availability of high marginal cost successful treatments, especially per life saved related to screening or diagnostic tests.

---

the demands of the *Patient's Charter*) the nature, extent, and quality of treatment available will change to meet those expectations.

The second area is where rationing is intimately bound up with service development. There will always be rationing at the "leading edge" of treatment whether or not a procedure is still regarded as a research topic. Examples include the development of new pharmaceutical and genetically engineered products, and new equipment technology, particularly that driven by computerised systems.

The third area in which rationing occurs is where the marginal costs of diagnosis or intervention become extremely high, for example, the cost per life saved as a result of a screening programme. A judgment must be taken on effectiveness grounds about whether a diagnostic test or treatment is appropriate, particularly for relatively infrequent conditions. In other words, rationing occurs where the cost of achieving a "true positive" diagnosis is considered unacceptably high.

Rationing semantics

By rationing, we mean any system or arrangement that delivers less care or treatment, or provides less physical support services, than would be considered ideal by an informed group of patients and healthcare professionals. No doubt every person has his or her own view of what is more or less important in the provision of healthcare. Some will argue that life saving procedures must be given priority for any funds; often such treatments could not, however, be given unless there was a building in which it could be provided, with suitably trained staff, who are aware of the latest evidence or the effectiveness of the care proposed, and with the necessary equipment in place to provide such care. Put another way, a discussion of rationing cannot focus only on medical, nursing, and related services immediate to a patient's healthcare needs.

Rationing covers all aspects of healthcare provision. Rationing the use of GP time for an individual consultation, as a result of the funding mechanisms for primary care, is just as much an aspect of rationing as reducing the availability of coronary artery bypass grafts for very elderly people with co-morbidities. Different reasons may be given for the decisions taken, and these may be more or less acceptable to those affected, but they are all rationing decisions. Attempting to side step the problem by emphasising clinical and cost effectiveness is disingenuous. Eventually a decision has to be taken about the level of effectiveness of a treatment below which that treatment will not be given. This implicitly rations that treatment, albeit perhaps on quite reasonable and relatively objective grounds.

Some people find the use of the term "rationing" uncomfortable. For them rationing is synonymous with cuts, with reductions, with insufficient amounts of care, and with the idea that unpalatable and tough decisions have to be taken. Undoubtedly, rationing is linked to the need for tough decisions, but rationing is also an ethical word. Rationing implies fair shares for all or, in healthcare, at least equal treatment for equal need. Rationing thus implies the principle of equity—that people will receive treatment appropriate to their clinical need with the most effective care available at the time. Conversely, terms such as "priority setting" and "resource allocation" do not of themselves imply equity. These are weasel words that provide a wide latitude to those making the decisions to steer resources to where *they* think services should be provided. It is not surprising, therefore, that politicians, health service managers, and clinicians have tried to avoid the term "rationing", but have been forced to be explicit that, within resource allocation decisions, the principle of equity—equal care for equal need—is of fundamental importance. Rationing implies and incorporates fair shares and just allocations.[2]

Although many politicians, and some managers and clinicians, seem embarrassed when the term is used, rationing is *not* a "dirty word". Those who oppose the idea that rationing is inevitable often appear to be arguing against using the word rationing rather than against what rationing implies. As we shall see in what follows, the sheer breadth and depth of those services that are not available at present within the UK National Health Service can only be described as rationing. "Rationing" should not be used in its pejorative sense, but rather in the positive recognition that when decisions must be taken they should be taken ethically and equitably. Rationing need not lead to defeatism, as some suggest,[3] but should rather be a spur to more efficient and effective care.

Underpinning assumptions

Much of this discussion of rationing makes a number of important assumptions. Some of these are not strictly borne out in current practice but support the contention that rationing is inevitable:

45

1 In the UK services are not, by and large, rationed by price. This is not true of dentistry and some pharmaceutical products for which prescription charges are levied. For most hospital and community health services and primary care, however, price is not a consideration as it is in some countries. Non-price rationing would still be required whether or not price rationing was involved.

2 Health care in the NHS will continue to be funded out of taxation. There are those who have suggested that, increasingly, other methods of funding will be needed. Whether or not they are right, the assumption made here is that rationing will be necessary regardless of whether the NHS remains publicly funded out of taxation and free at the point of delivery. Although there is a dynamic budget for healthcare and the ceiling has some flexibility, nevertheless it is and will remain insufficient to remove the need for rationing. Rationing does not begin only when non-tax based funding is introduced.

3 Technological advances will continue to occur on many fronts although some expensive surgical techniques will become obsolete as a result of developments in gene therapy and molecular biology; the explosive growth in the development of new treatments will continue to put significant pressure on healthcare budgets.

These assumptions suggest that those who are reluctant to engage in a debate on rationing believe that: (1) society will vote sufficient funds (via taxation or in some other way) to obviate the need for tough decisions on those forms and types of treatment that are provided; (2) there are sufficient resources to pay for technological development and that, as some services become obsolete and cease, more efficient and effective treatments will be discovered; or (3) there are so many inefficiencies in present provision and so many treatments that are unnecessary or ineffective, that if they were removed there would be sufficient money to fund all other elements of care.

None of these three views or beliefs can be sustained. Substantial increases in public funding of the NHS is highly unlikely and not economically feasible. Technological advance will continue rapidly and will require increasingly sophisticated staff and equipment with associated costs of training and development. Cutting out inefficient and non-effective treatments is somewhat more promising because there is no doubt that inefficiencies and some non-effective treatments remain. The identification of such inefficiencies and non-effective treatments of itself, however, takes resources. Additional research is needed to identify those areas of care that are either inefficient or insufficiently effective, and ways then have to be found to stop them happening. More challenging is the difficulty of identifying those treatments and interventions for which outcome measures are either non-existent or difficult to obtain, but where those involved believe that the intervention or treatment is beneficial in some way. Efforts must also be made to reduce the considerable variance between hospitals in the application of procedures and intervention.[4]

The Anti-Rationing Group suggests five categories, within which significant savings might be made, and which would eradicate the need for rationing.[10] These are

- identifying inappropriate expenditure, that is, care that would be paid for by other agencies
- imprecisely specified services
- care for which effectiveness is insufficiently justified
- "over-purchasing"
- paying too high a price for care.

They go on to suggest that "it is inhuman and financially indefensible to propose rationing while there is ill-founded spending. . .". This general contention is superficially attractive but ultimately misleading, although some gains can undoubtedly be achieved by reducing waste through volume reductions and price controls. It is misleading for two reasons: first, the savings achieved, even at the inflated levels suggested when set against cost pressures in the NHS, will not be sufficient to eliminate rationing; second, and more importantly, the proposals are in themselves simply rationing by another name—cost shifting onto other agencies (which may or may not have the resources either), or reducing expenditure on services for which effectiveness is not yet proven, or establishing 'reasonable' thresholds for treatments on a marginal cost per life saved basis. What the group has done, helpfully, is to provide a good foundation for rationing!

An example of the difficulties of basing rationing decisions on clearcut outcome measures can be seen in the provision of health visiting to young parents and their babies. Health visitors have an important role in preventing poor parenting practice and in encouraging good nutrition and infant development. Often health visitors identify incipient problems, ranging from a lack of confidence in a young parent through the whole range of experience to potential child abuse. The "craft" aspects of a health visitor's role, as in many other branches of nursing, is often overlooked or undervalued. Determining the level of resources required to provide sufficient numbers of health visitors with appropriate training and experience, for a defined population, is a judgment that professional staff must take partly on the funds available and partly on the availability of suitably trained staff. Cutting back of health visiting implies a tolerance of discrimination, especially towards disadvantaged parents.

What is the cost of a life saved by early identification of possible physical or sexual abuse; the cost of lower attainment later in life as a result of poor nutrition early in infancy; the cost of stress to young parents of infant illnesses and the psychological damage that this may do to the family, not to mention the later cost to the NHS in physical and psychological care? These, and many other aspects of care that good health visiting will identify, are difficult if not impossible to quantify. Those who argue that treatments should only be provided if clear outcome measures can be offered are rejecting professional expertise as a guide to necessary resource allocation.

A similar situation can be seen on the wards of many hospitals. The steady reduction in the numbers of trained nursing staff able to sit with, counsel, or advise seriously ill patients reduces the quality of both the patient and the nursing experience. Surely it is rationing when patients, as a result of tight staffing at nights in many of our hospitals, die alone in side wards? Surely it is rationing that many hospitals can only manage with agency nursing staff who are not part of the regular ward team? The agency staff member may ensure that the quantity of absolutely necessary care is provided, but the level of agency staffing may reduce the overall quality of care to the patients, as well as introducing inefficiencies into the working of the ward. Many staff work for agencies because there is a shortage of appropriately trained staff in all parts of the NHS, one reason being the relatively poor pay for staff with substantial skills gained over many years of committed and dedicated work.

Bringing wage levels, staffing levels, and training availability up to a level that many would agree is necessary might not be considered by some as related to rationing. The cost could, in broad terms, be calculated relatively easily; but it is another aspect of rationing nevertheless, and would be yet one more significant pressure for additional resources in an already overextended system. The ARG has calculated that the NHS might save perhaps 20% by reducing what it perceives as potentially ineffective community nursing and other provisions. As the discussion above noted, this calculation is highly contentious. On the other side of the balance sheet, disregarding technological advances and the many areas of present rationing within the NHS (see below), a 10% increase in staffing levels for doctors, nurses, and paramedical staff, and a 10% increase in the salary of those staff, would alone add £6 billion to the cost of the NHS. When this is added to all the other pressures, some of which are described later, even a 20% saving would be insufficient to make rationing unnecessary. The possible cost savings from abolishing the internal market pale into insignificance.

Rationing: common themes and specific services

Rationing within the NHS can be considered in two ways: first, by consideration of rationing features that are common to most or all aspects of healthcare, and, second, within individual specialty areas or related service provision.

Common themes

A number of common themes can be discerned that influence the way in which decisions are made on the availability of resources to different areas of healthcare. The first of these is an implicit, and sometimes explicit, calculation of the cost of a life saved as a result of some intervention or other. This is seen particularly in health economic calculations of decisions on screening. Cholesterol screening to reduce heart disease provides a good example of the high marginal cost of additional quality adjusted life years (QALYs) which might be gained. One study compared two alternatives. The first is to promote healthy eating in the general population (the population approach); the second is the same but in combination with general practitioner screening for high cholesterol levels, followed by dietary treatment for those in the relevant range. Donaldson[6] shows that the population approach alone generates 3800 QALYs at a cost of only £10 per QALY; whereas the screening and treatment programme would be extremely expensive but generate only an additional 400 QALYs at a marginal cost of £100,000 per QALY. It is clear that additional benefit could be achieved but at such a cost that it is not a practical proposition.

Similar calculations have been done for breast cancer screening, which inter-alia, compute the marginal cost of a tumour detected by widening the age criteria for standard screening programmes (at present 50–65 years of age). For example screening women in the age range 40–49 annually rather than at two yearly intervals would reduce mortality by around 20 per cent.[7] Both these examples demonstrate how extra statistical lives are *always* there to be saved, but at unaffordable costs.

Political considerations are an ever present feature of rationing within healthcare. The past decade has seen a steady increase in our understanding of quality enhancement and risk management in health services. Economies of scale are essential up to some optimum of throughput. The quality of surgical operations improves the more skilled the surgeon and the more frequently he or she undertakes that operation. Support for junior staff, particularly out of hours, demands a sufficiently large staff team, which in turn requires fewer more intensively staffed units, but which are clinically safer and provide higher quality care.

Yet public and political demands for the retention of small district general hospitals often conflict with the steady development of technology and the need for appropriate training support and accreditation of staff, and militates against an improvement in clinical safety—unless additional resources are provided. Perversely rationing occurs as a result of overprovision! Too many resources are put into infrastructure and management costs of too many units which are unable to provide the higher quality care and the economies of scale necessary. Whether retaining small units is a sensible decision or not, it is nevertheless a feature of the way in which rationing occurs, and will continue to occur. Who is to say that local people are not right in wanting 'easy local access and availability of care? Health professionals take one view, largely as a response to cost containment pressures. Local health service users understandably take another and different view.

It is hopeless to suggest that, in some ideal world, all services would be in the right place provided by staff who are fully trained in the latest technology and are all working at the leading edge of practice. Emphasising clinical effectiveness is essential, but given the pace at which technology is moving it is unrealistic to believe that every doctor or other healthcare professional will be working to the same standards and able to encompass latest thinking at all times. Indeed this may even be dangerous. Sometimes new techniques are found to be less attractive than first thought: a new drug, which may have been heavily marketed and which is thought to provide a breakthrough in treatment, is found to have unacceptable and unforeseen side effects. Without trial and error, we will never discover new products that will treat disease and prolong life, but medicine and healthcare do not move forward in discrete fully described steps which can be disseminated quickly and easily to all involved. Health care is by its very nature a "fuzzy" science, and it is therefore appropriate that some new techniques are rationed until they are proven, and some will remain rationed as a result of cost–benefit studies on the effectiveness of the treatment and on agreed thresholds for admission to a treatment programme.

It is perfectly correct to describe this as rationing. These services are appropriately rationed for good reason. Diversion of the argument on to a discussion of clinical effectiveness is not to suggest an alternative to rationing. Rather, discussions of clinical effectiveness and the way in which this informs decisions on who will or will not be treated are part of the "due process" of rationing. A proper focus on cost–benefit analysis and clinical effectiveness of care, rooted in a culture of evidence based medicine, enables rationing decisions to be made as objectively as possible, ensuring that all elements of the calculation are explicit and available openly for scrutiny.

The well documented case of Jaymee Bowen (Child B) provides a clear example of rationing in practice.[5,9] She was denied a *second* bone marrow transplantation (BMT) on the clinical grounds that the chance of success was, perhaps, 2%, and the probable balance of harms and benefits to her was not encouraging. The cost would have been in the region of £75 000. After the unduly publicised court case, she did not receive a bone marrow transplantation but instead an experimental treatment—donor lymphocyte infusion—which was ultimately unsuccessful.

The decision to withhold the BMT treatment was a rationing decision made on good clinical grounds, but which also saved a substantial amount of money. The question that this raised—and one that no one has yet realistically sought to answer—is what clinicians and the public would consider to be a price worth paying (in money and potential harms to the patient) for a small probability of success. Even a one in a million chance of success would be considered if the treatment cost was only say, £1, or £10, or perhaps £100. But £1000, or £10 000, or £100 000? Somewhere there is a breakpoint; at some level, through clinicians and health service managers, and ultimately politicians, we must accept that, *as a rule* (a rule that may, for good reason, sometimes be broken), the health service will not pay more than some (large) sum, for a poor (say, < 1%; 0·1%?) prognosis of success.

Rationing by price, waiting list, geographical access, or other mechanism occurs widely. Sometimes such rationing is beneficial in reducing the moral hazard associated with a service that is free at the point of delivery. Any service that appears free may be abused in its use. Price hurdles, such as those found in primary care in the USA, *can* under some circumstances assist in managing demand and ensuring that patients use the service only when they consider it essential. Such price hurdles also put some patients off using a service when they ought to be receiving care and has the effect of denying care to those on low incomes or those who have other disadvantages. The introduction of charges for eye tests in the UK has evidently reduced access for many people which in turn has reduced the screening potential for diabetes and glaucoma. Not only is this a very explicit form of rationing, but would cost a considerable amount to re-provide through state funding. Similarly NHS dentistry for adults is now more or less restricted to those on welfare benefits and a lucky few who have been with the same dentist for some years or who are able to find a dentist prepared to continue to provide care with NHS funding. The particular financial mechanisms and rules that prohibit co-payments within dentistry have ensured that rationing is an endemic feature of dental care, although rationing would still be inevitable if co-payments were introduced. If, on the other hand, universal free-at-point-of-use dentistry was reintroduced, it would be immensely costly and there would still be a need to ration by non-price means. There is no escape.

One problem in determining the extent of rationing within healthcare is in drawing the boundary of what is appropriately healthcare free at the point of delivery funded out of taxation and properly provided by the NHS, and what might be termed "health related care" provided by other agencies (as Roberts and colleagues[10] also note). This debate has found its clearest focus in the argument between the NHS and Social Service Departments of local authorities over what constitutes health care and what constitutes social care. At one point this debate turned on what became amusingly known as the "social bath"—when should the NHS pay for a community nurse to bathe an elderly person in his or her own home free as a healthcare service, or when should this be the responsibility of the local authority with the power and local discretion to make a charge. The dispute was over the extent to which a community nurse or other healthcare aide would be able to use the period of bathing to check on the health of the person and to provide preventive advice.

Most health authorities and local authorities have now agreed on criteria for funding of residential and continuing care provision, and have moved beyond squabbles over detailed boundary problems. Nevertheless there remain some intractable and growing difficulties in the distinction between continued nursing home provision with a health element, and residential care provision in which the healthcare element is contained within general medical service funding of local GPs. As the population becomes increasingly elderly and frail, the distinction between health and social care becomes ever more blurred. One effect of this is to encourage a debate, fostered by the BMA and the General Medical Services Committee, of what is known as "core services" provided by GPs.

Most health authorities at the time of writing are in negotiation with GPs locally to determine payments for those elements of care provided by them to residential and nursing homes, which go beyond the basic requirements of the GP contract. The probable outcome is a constraint on the quantity of care that health authorities will be prepared to purchase over and above the GP contract. In other words, the effect is a more explicit form of rationing of the levels of care being provided in the community, with implications for relocation of some forms of secondary care and the quality of life for residents. At its most basic, this may mean some residents having to go into hospital for periods of time when they might otherwise have been able to remain at the residential or nursing home.

Health promotion and preventive strategies provide another unclear boundary between NHS healthcare and personal responsibility. By and large the NHS does not pay for leisure facilities that may improve fitness, although there are moves in some areas to enable GPs to "prescribe" structured exercise programmes. Health promotion units provide advice on nutrition, sexual health, drug abuse, parenting skills, and so forth, and may offer advice, guidance, and information materials. Rarely do health promotion activities extend to payments to encourage healthy lifestyles, even though these might reduce costs on the health service in the long term. Some national systems pay for a wider range of homoeopathic and complementary medical care than the UK. Visits to spas, provision of traditional medicines, and chiropractic care are all heavily rationed within the NHS.

At a yet further remove from traditional healthcare, both health authorities and local authorities have a vested interest in reducing accidents, especially childhood accidents in the home and road traffic accidents. Health authorities are not empowered to support local authorities in physical arrangements for traffic quieting, for example, road humps ("sleeping policemen") and road narrowing, even though these might save substantial cost to the NHS "downstream". Is this supply rationing by another name? As we saw earlier, the pressure to reduce community nursing costs may well have an effect in increasing childhood accidents if young parents are not given sufficient advice from appropriately trained staff on how to minimise the likelihood of accidents in the home, especially accidental self-poisoning in infants. All these examples of restricting or redefining the boundary of the NHS do not mean that rationing is eliminated; it will simply be shifted to other agencies.

There are thus a number of "cross cutting themes" which demonstrate the extent of rationing in most areas of healthcare provision. Some of these are not unreasonable, and decisions will always have to be taken about the appropriate agency for providing some form of care, and the budget available for that care. What these themes demonstrate, however, is the sheer extent of rationing in the NHS and thus its inevitability in the foreseeable future.

Examples of rationing in specialty areas

In this section we further illustrate the general case made above by analysing rationing in specialty areas. It should become clear that exhausting the potential healthcare benefits in these areas is beyond current, or any reasonable projection, of available resources. Dentistry and optometry are two ready examples of care that is rationed explicitly. Continuing care to residential and nursing home users has been squeezed; health authorities have had to draw back from providing measures to prevent accidental and non-accidental injury to children; salary and infrastructure cost pressures within the service demonstrate not only a rationing of skill and expertise, but identify the size of investment needed if the deficits are to be addressed. Such an investment is highly unlikely.

Obstetric care

Most areas of the NHS suffer from some form of rationing, although it is not always easy to demonstrate a link between the availability of care and the outcome of treatment. Prenatal obstetric care, for example, is rationed significantly. "Changing Childbirth" has placed an emphasis on team midwifery and on ensuring that women receive continuity of care from a small defined group of midwives. Yet it is still true that the amount of prenatal support is inadequate and that many women do not see a consultant obstetrician at any stage during pregnancy. For many women this may not be absolutely essential, although it can be argued plausibly that some difficulties in pregnancy and at term might be eliminated or ameliorated by wider availability of consultants and easier access to antenatal care.

GP consultations

Similarly, within general practice, the time for consultation is strictly limited by the number of patients each GP is required to enlist, which in turn is a function of the remuneration formula for general practice. The average GP list is around 2000 patients. In some areas of lower morbidity, a GP may be able to provide care to a larger group of patients, whereas in urban areas and sparse rural areas lists will be shorter. The size of list determines the demand on the GP, and sets limits on the length of consultation, the ease with which the GP is able to undertake home visits, and the amount of time for involvement in continuing medical education. All of these have a bearing on service quality, a quality that is strictly rationed by the funding mechanism. Halving the GP list size would provide much better opportunities for a higher quality care to patients but at a significant cost to the Exchequer.

To suggest that this is not a significant form of rationing would be perverse, but does beg the question of what is an optimum primary care service, and on what basis the parameters of that service are decided. The optimum consultation period will vary from GP to GP and from practice to practice; the level of referral for diagnostic tests at the local hospital will vary from practice to practice; the level of out of hours provision and the extent to which GPs undertake their own out of hours calls will also vary. What is not at issue is that the average "wage" for the GP is considerably lower than that for hospital consultants, that working hours are relatively long, and that the opportunities for active involvement in the planning and management of care, and in continuing professional and medical education, are relatively poor.

Recent emphasis on encouraging research and development activity in general practice is to be welcomed, but is yet another pressure on overstretched GPs (and other primary care contractors). The time for such activity will have to be carved out of an already busy schedule. It is unclear whether the outcomes of care are lower than they would be if GPs had more time to spend with patients or were able to order, for example, more diagnostic tests. Overall costs to the service *might* not increase if the improvements in primary care and early detection of morbidity led to reduced treatment costs. Conversely, early identification of problems may well mean more treatment rather than less, patients being treated more quickly for more ailments, and overall living longer; the screw of rationing is tightened yet again.

54

Mental health

Mental health care provides perhaps the most obvious example of rationing at present. All elements of mental health care are heavily constrained and in many cases woefully inadequate. Child and adolescent psychiatry is underdeveloped and, in many areas, community child mental health services are poorly resourced and do not include all those specialist components of the multidisciplinary team that good practice would dictate. Adolescent psychiatry is under-resourced especially for late adolescents who have severe psychotic disorders. Many of these young people are treated inappropriately on adult inpatient acute admission wards. Similarly, adult acute services are themselves under tremendous pressure, often running at over 100% occupancy. Services for mentally disordered offenders are insufficient both in the number of places and in the range of therapies available. Mental health care for elderly people, especially community nursing and multidisciplinary locally accessible care, is underprovided. The cost of achieving sufficient care in all of these areas is huge, and different organisations have made varying estimates ranging up to an additional £2 billion for a fully functioning service. Even this, however, does not imply that *all* benefits which a mental health service might confer have been exhausted.

Whatever the cost of providing an effective service, there is absolutely no doubt among those who provide mental health care that it is heavily rationed both within and between subspecialties. Counselling and psychological therapies perhaps fare worst and there appears to be real discrimination among health authorities in funding psychotherapeutic treatment. Clinical psychology is underprovided in most areas, and what should be multidisciplinary teams often comprise largely nurses with some psychiatric support. None of this argues against careful analysis of what staff do with patients and a requirement to obtain information on outcomes of care. Much greater emphasis on outcome measures is needed, and on research and development programmes that ensure that evidence of effectiveness is utilised. Psychiatry seems to suffer more than most specialties from a reluctance to learn from work done in other areas. The "not invented here" syndrome only encourages further rationing, and mental health care is no exception.

Mental health care provides some of the best illustrations of where the extension of evidence based care would improve quality but at a cost that almost certainly would not be recouped from efficiency gains elsewhere. Family interventions (restraint of high expressed emotion), rapid crisis response, and assertive outreach are all techniques that improve the quality of care, and support and sustain patients in community settings; the deployment costs are, however, higher than potential savings on inpatient care.

Even if all services were to do their best to apply good practice from elsewhere, the widely documented under-resourcing of current provision suggests a substantial rationing of care to service users. The apparent increase in the number of homicides and serious offences committed by mentally disordered offenders may be more apparent than real, but suggests unacceptable levels of continuing support to and supervision of mentally ill people in community settings. Policy developments of the 1970s and 1980s, notably the emphasis on community mental health care to replace the large institutions, has not been matched by the funds necessary to provide a dispersed community oriented service. Managing such a service is far more challenging than managing single institutions, even though the abuses that were uncovered in some of those institutions in the 1960s and 1970s demonstrated a lack of management there too. The neglect of patients in the community is an obvious example of the present rationing of care compounded by a lack of emphasis on the management of mental health services and the need for funds to match policy imperatives.

Cardiovascular disease

The last example concerns one of the chief killers of the twentieth century—coronary artery disease. Reducing incidence of myocardial infarction (heart attack) and resultant death or disability would require heightened investment in health promotion (notably anti-smoking and diet), mobile coronary care units, rapid response systems, and improved availability of early therapeutic interventions. One small aspect of this—thrombolytic therapy—deserves some attention because it demonstrates most clearly the dilemma of rationing posed by the available evidence of treatment efficiency.[11] Without a detailed excursion into the literature, it is sufficient to note that recent studies have shown strong, but not overwhelming, evidence of the benefits of early thrombolytic injection after a heart attack.[12] It is unclear whether health authorities and fundholders should demand (purchase) rapid availability of this therapy for *all* patients, or accept that a more selective policy may lead to the death of a few patients who might have died anyway. The cost of a comprehensive uniform service places a very high marginal value on the (few) lives saved. In other words, saving the "last" life is unaffordable.

Conclusions

The discussion presented here has sought to demonstrate two interrelated points: first, that rationing is inevitable given present and likely future NHS funding; and second, that attempts to deny that rationing exists or will continue to exist are either misleading or self defeating, in that they are simply further forms of rationing. Many other examples could have been given to illustrate the argument.

The need to ration services does not imply any lessening in demands for more resources for the NHS, or suggest that the NHS should be anything other than funded out of taxation and be free at the point of delivery. The inevitability of rationing should not be a brake on progress, but rather a spur to identifying genuinely inappropriate care, reducing unnecessary variance and production inefficiencies, and eliminating proven ineffectiveness. These are landable aims, but they will not remove the need for rationing. Rather they will ensure that rationing is objective, explicit, and equitable.

This chapter has considered *why* rationing is inevitable, not how effective rationing (priority setting and resource allocation) can be achieved. That is covered elsewhere (for example, by Honigsbaum et al.[13]). It is worth noting, however, that the challenging, uncomfortable, and sometimes unacceptable rationing processes from elsewhere—for example, Oregon or New Zealand—should not divert attention from the need for some process that enables society to manage adequately the hard reality and inevitability of resource scarcity. As Maynard[14] has suggested, whether the term "rationing" is used or some other gentler word, the consequences of rationing require open and honest debate.

1 New B (Rationing Agenda Group). *The rationing agenda in the NHS*. London: King's Fund, 1996.
2 Doyal L. Needs, rights and equity: moral quality in healthcare rationing, *Qual Health Care* 1995;4:273–83.
3 Mullen P. *Is healthcare rationing really necessary?* Birmingham: HSMC, 1995.
4 Andersen FT, Mooney G. *The challenges of medical practice variations*. Basingstoke: MacMillan, 1990.
5 Entwistle VA, Watt SI, Bradbury R, Lesley JP. Media coverage of the Child B case. *BMJ* 1996;312:1587–91.
6 Donaldson C. Using economics to assess the place of screening. *J Med Screening* 1994;1: 124–9.
7 Tabar L, Fagerberg G, Chan HH, Duffy SW, Gad A. Screening for breast cancer in women aged under 50: mode of detection incidence, fatality and histology. *J Med Screening* 1995;2:94–8.
8 Klein R, Day P, Redmayne S. *Managing scarcity—priority setting and rationing in the NHS* Buckingham: Open University Press, 1996.
9 Barclay S. *Jaymee: the story of Child B*. London: Viking, 1996.
10 Roberts C, Crosby D, Grundy P, et al. The wasted millions. *HSJ*, 10 October, 1996.
11 York University. *Asprin and myocardial infarction*. York: NHS Centre for Reviews and Dissemination, 1995:1.
12 Rawles J. Magnitude of benefit from earlier thrombolytic treatment in acute myocardial infarction: new evidence from Grampian region early anistreplase trial. *BMJ* 1996;312: 212–16.
13 Honigsbaum F, Calltorp J, Ham C, Holmström S: *Priority setting processes for healthcare*. Oxford: Radcliffe Press, 1995.
14 Maynard A. Rationing health care. *BMJ* 1996;313:1499.

5 What does the public think about rationing? A review of the evidence

JACK KNEESHAW

What does the public think of health care rationing? Does it think it necessary, or does it believe that the National Health Service (NHS) should provide all the treatment that patients need? If the public does think that rationing is necessary, to what forms of treatment or care would it give priority? Does it believe in heroic efforts to keep people alive, or does it favour treatments to relieve pain and suffering? Is it prejudiced against mental health? Does it believe that some sorts of people, say young or old people, should gain priority access to treatment? And who does it think should be responsible for rationing? Doctors? Managers? Politicians? Or the public itself? The purpose of this chapter is to review the available evidence on these questions.

There are a number of reasons for considering the public's attitudes to questions of rationing. First, Government policy has explicitly stressed the importance of allowing the public to shape the debate about patient care. The *Patient's Charter*[1] and the NHS Management Executive's publication, *Local Voices*,[2] have both recommended that district health authorities involve "interested" groups (local people, general practitioners, health care providers, etc.) in the decisions over which health services should be purchased.[3]

Second, incidents such as the Child B case, where there appeared to be a denial of treatment for a particular individual, have sparked off considerable public reaction. It is clear that, when it comes to particular cases like that of Child B, the public often has an intense and personal reaction to the tragic situations of individuals. But does this reaction translate into anything coherent when asked to consider the issues, not in relation to a particular individual, but as a matter of policy?

Third, democracy needs public debate and understanding if it is to function properly. Finding out what the public knows and where it stands

58

Table 5.1   Main sources of evidence on public opinion and healthcare rationing

Methodology	
Survey: national	MORI, 1993
	Gallup, 1994
	OPCS Omnibus, 1995
Survey: local	Bath, 1990
	Colchester, 1991
	City and Hackney, 1992
	East Surrey, 1992
	Salford, 1992
Public meeting	Cambridge and Huntingdon, 1996
Community group	City and Hackney, 1992
	East Surrey, 1992
Focus group	Salford, 1992
	Bromley, 1994
	Somerset, 1995
Health forum	Mid-Essex, 1991
Citizens' jury	Cambridge and Huntingdon, 1996

is the first step in trying to see how the quality of public debate can be raised.

Against this background, this chapter seeks to answer a number of questions. First, what sources of evidence are there to tell us what the public view on healthcare rationing is? Second, does this evidence consist exclusively of survey data or are there other sources of information that may help define public opinion? Third, what problems are there in using this evidence? Fourth, what does this evidence tell us about public opinion on health care rationing? And fifth, what are the implications of these findings for the public's role in the process of prioritising?

Eliciting public views on healthcare rationing

A number of different methods have been used to elicit public views on healthcare rationing. These range from undertaking surveys to analysing the decisions taken, or views expressed, by community groups, focus groups, citizens' juries, and public meetings. Each method is prone to deliver its own "view" of what constitutes public opinion on matters relating to the NHS and the rationing debate in particular.

Surveys: postal and interview, national and local

Most of the evidence on British public opinion and health care rationing comes from surveys undertaken within the past five years (Table 5.1). These surveys have been based on both postal and interview questionnaires, and have taken place at both the local and the national level. Although the evidence gathered from such surveys is probably the most obvious place to start an analysis of public views on health care rationing, there are several problems inherent in transposing opinions expressed in surveys into what can be termed a "public view".

The first is the problem of question design and wording. Poorly or ambiguously worded questions can lead to inconsistent responses. Respondents may give views that are incompatible, may not understand the question being asked, or may answer two questions that are designed to elicit the same response in a very different manner (if, for example, one question contains more information than another). This leads to a second difficulty with survey data, namely that respondents' views on health care may change with knowledge.[4] This can bring into question the validity of some survey data and may cause opinions or preferences to lack stability. As a consequence, those questioning the quality of survey evidence have pointed out that it can often provide "simple and superficial" information.[5]

Another criticism levelled at survey evidence on healthcare rationing is that respondents' own experiences tend to be different to the hypothetical questions posed.[4] In other words, the questions posed do not relate to "real life" issues as experienced by the respondents, and it can be difficult for them to think as they would if they were actually faced with the question in reality. Finally, it ought to be remembered that poor and unrepresentative response rates pose a problem in the use of survey data. Low response rates in inner city areas have certainly been a problem in at least one local survey, as has been the difficulty of gauging the opinions of minority groups from small samples of the population.[6]

Community groups, focus groups, and citizens' juries

Other methods, apart from large scale surveys, can be used either to supplement the survey data or to offset its shortcomings. Among these, the use of evidence obtained from community groups, focus groups, and citizens' juries has been gaining in popularity.

Community groups, focus groups, and citizens' juries differ from surveys as each is the result of a more deliberative style of opinion polling. All three rely on removing a small section of the population and placing them in an environment where there is access to some degree of information and where decisions may be "talked through". In the case of community groups, the sample of the population is made up of community leaders and local figures of responsibility, chosen as the community's "representatives". Focus groups and citizens' juries, by contrast, are usually selected to be demographically representative of the local population. However, the fundamental approach is the same as that for the community group. A "representative" selection of the local population is taken aside and exposed to information that will help to shape their views. Groups can then deliberate over the decisions, ask questions of experts, and spend time formulating considered opinions rather than "thinking on the spot" as respondents to surveys are generally expected to do.

Nevertheless, evidence from such groups provides us with at least two problems: first, group deliberation presents us with the problem of group dynamics—it may be that some members of the group are able to dominate the discussions at the expense of others; second, evidence from these examples of deliberative democracy is in short supply. We have evidence from only two series of community group studies, three series of focus groups, one citizens' jury, and one "forum" that fails to fall neatly into any of these categories (see Table 5.1). In short, this method of eliciting public opinion remains at an experimental stage. This method has so far been little used and its benefits and drawbacks have, therefore, been difficult to establish.

Public meetings

Another methodology has seen evidence from public meetings used to help constitute a "public view" on healthcare rationing. This methodology is primarily used as a means of supporting evidence, often qualitative in approach, picking up on statements made by members of the public, or picking up on a "general feeling". In Britain, at least one such meeting has been called in the Cambridge and Huntingdon Health Authority (1996). It did, however, suffer from a condition common to such meetings—namely "volunteer bias"[5], that is, those attending the meeting were, for the most part, made up of interested parties such as patients' groups or health care workers. As a consequence, using evidence from public meetings to uncover a "public" view is an activity that should be undertaken with caution. For this reason—and because evidence from this particular methodology is so scarce—we rely on it only very briefly in the following sections.

Is rationing necessary?

Having looked at the *sources* of evidence of public opinion on healthcare rationing, we can now move on to an *analysis* of the available evidence. This will be done in four stages, each stage looking at the public's view on a particular question. To begin with we will look at the question of whether health care rationing is perceived by the public to be necessary (Table 5.2).

The evidence that deals with this question is scarce, and on first inspection seems contradictory. Almost all the evidence comes from national survey

Table 5.2 Public views on the necessity of rationing

Year	Methodology	Statement	Agree (%)	Don't know (%)
1991	National survey, Gallup	**Everyone should have all the health care they need no matter how much it costs**	77	5
		There is no end to the demand for health care, and health care must therefore compete for funds with education, pensions, and other public services	18	
1993	National survey, MORI: $n=$ 2012	**Do you think that the NHS should have unlimited finding?**	51	7
		Or do you think that budgets should be set even if it means that some treatments will have higher priority than others?	42	
1994 (Aug)	National survey, Gallup: $n=$ 1027	**The NHS will always be able to provide everyone with every treatment they need**	16	5
		The NHS will always have to work out priorities so that some types of treatment and patients are given higher priority than others	79	

Sources: Gallup 29.10.91–5.11.91; Heginbotham,[7] MORI 1993; Gallup 9.8.94–15.8.94.

data, with only a small amount of qualitative evidence to tell us how the public would respond to this question when exposed to greater information in a focus group or citizens' jury. The three different quantitative measures on the subject also provide us with three different views. Almost certainly this results from the fact that the evidence in our possession has been gathered from surveys where subtle changes in question wording mean that none of the data we have are strictly comparable. As a result, eliciting a public view on the necessity of rationing is a tricky process. If we consider the three survey measures together, for a moment, the confusion becomes apparent.

Ostensibly, each poll deals with the central notion of whether the NHS should be able to undertake any treatment no matter what the cost. In the most recent poll (1994), only 16% of the respondents appeared to agree that the NHS had such a commitment (that is, 79% felt that some form of priority setting was inevitable). However, the earlier Gallup poll appears to have come to the opposite conclusion. There, 77% agreed that "everyone should have all the health care they need no matter how much it costs". The two views appear incompatible: one cannot have all the health care needed, *regardless of cost*, if the NHS "will always have to work out priorities so that some types of treatment and some patients are given higher priority than others". To confuse matters further, the views of the public in the MORI poll fall somewhere between the two Gallup indicators. There, public opinion is roughly divided equally (51–42) between those thinking that the NHS should benefit from unlimited funding and those believing that budgets should be set. In short, each poll seems to tell a different story. Is it possible to reconcile these differences?

One possible explanation involves the difference in question wording. The most recent poll (1994) asks the public a *factual* question (that is, which statement is true?), whereas the previous two polls (1991 and 1993) are based on *normative* responses (that is, what should be?). In other words, the polls are not tapping the same public attitudes. This is a common problem in the comparison of survey data and would suggest that each measure be read in isolation. If this is the case we might say that the public believes that rationing in the NHS *is a reality* (Gallup 1994) but that *it need not be* (Gallup 1991 and MORI 1993).

Another, quite different, explanation is that we may be observing a dramatic sea change in public opinion on healthcare rationing, perhaps a realisation on the public's behalf that there can be no such thing as "unlimited funding". The evidence to support this—which is tenuous given the fact that we have data from only three polls where the questions posed were not identical—is that the polls can be analysed chronologically. If we take this approach, an argument can be made which suggests that between 1991 and 1994 public opinion on the inevitability of health care rationing switched very quickly from "unrealistic" (that is, "everyone should have all the health care they need no matter how much it costs") to a position which could be said to be "realistic" (that is, "the NHS will always have to work out priorities").

Given the dearth of comparable data, however, this can only be a hypothesis. To many, it will also be regarded as highly implausible and somewhat mischievous. Changes in public opinion as dramatic as this are rare. It may be that such an explanation is simply "clutching at straws" and that the importance of changes in question wording is more important. Certainly, the small amount of qualitative evidence available from a local survey and a local focus group fails to offer a conclusive answer. The results from the survey showed that there was a "lack of acceptance that prioritisation should be necessary",[8] whereas the evidence from the Bromley focus group studies showed that "there was a general awareness and support for a finite budget for health care".[9] Whatever the case, the lack of data on this question—and the lack of evidence from the more focused methodologies—means that it is difficult to say with any certainty what the public's view on the necessity of rationing is.

What treatments are priorities?

The key to the rationing debate is deciding what ought to be prioritised. On this question, there is a reasonable amount of evidence—both from survey data and group decision making—to tell us what the public thinks. To make analysis more straightforward we have split this evidence into two sections. First, we analyse the public's position on the prioritisation of *services* or *treatments*. Second, we examine whether the public feels that certain *people* ought to be prioritised or whether some groups of patients deserve to have a lower priority for treatment than others.*

Most measures of the public's attitudes towards prioritising treatments can be split into one of two categories. The first of these is made up of those measures that ask the public to rank *specific* services or treatments (Tables 5.3–5.5). In the second category the public are asked to agree or disagree with a more *general* policy statement (Table 5.6) or to rank *types* of treatment (Table 5.7).

Tables 5.3 and 5.4 belong to the former category. Both compare the rankings of the public with doctors, hospital consultants, and managers. We have separated the two tables simply because the treatments prioritised in each are different. Nevertheless, it is clear even from a cursory analysis that both tables tell us much the same thing.

To begin with, it is reasonably clear that the doctors, consultants, and managers polled held broadly similar views. This we take to be "professional" or "expert" opinion. For the public, it is also clear that they too held broadly consistent opinions. Priority rankings vary only slightly between the two measures of public opinion in Table 5.3 and the two measures of public opinion in Table 5.4. In Table 5.3, for instance, both measures of public opinion ranked treatments for children with life threatening illnesses as the top priority, with care for the dying as second. Preventive services (such as screening for breast cancer) also scored highly (ranked 4 and 3). Further down the list, a similar consistency is evident, with disagreements over the priority accorded to the use of high technology surgery (ranked 3 and 7) and community services (9 and 5) the only notable exceptions.

Table 5.4 shows a similar story. All treatment rankings were within two places of each other. It also seems that, as in Table 5.3, consistency in ranking was most defined at the top and bottom of the rankings. Both indicators of public opinion rated childhood immunisation, care offered by GPs, and screening for breast cancer highly, with treatment for schizophrenia and cancer treatment for smokers given the lowest priority.

This consistency was evident in another local survey where the question wording was different but close enough to be comparable. In East Surrey,

---

* This separation of priorities for *treatments* and priorities for *patients* is by no means perfect. Most treatments can also be seen as a service for a category of patient (for example "treatment for AIDS" may be seen to be similar to services for "people who are terminally ill") Nevertheless, a separation does exist. Ranking treatments that preserve quality of life over life saving interventions, for instance, does not involve much of a judgement of on the category of patient. For this reason, we distinguish between priorities for treatments and patients while acknowledging that an overlap between these cateogries exists.

Table 5.3 Priority rating of specific health services: public and expert opinion

Services or treatments	Public, City and Hackney (1992): $n =$ 335	Public, OPCS Omnibus (1995): $n =$ 1975	General Practitioners, City and Hackney (1992): $n = 66$	Consultants, City and Hackney (1992): $n =$ 116
Treatments for children with life threatening illness (leukaemia)	1	1	5	2
Special care and pain relief for people who are dying (hospice care)	2	2	4	4
High technology surgery and procedures which treat life threatening conditions (heart transplants)	3	7	9	9
Preventive services (screening, immunisation)	4	3	6	7
Surgery to help people with disabilities carry out everyday tasks (hip replacements)	5	4	7	5
Services for people with mental illness (psychiatric wards)	6	6	2	1
Intensive care for premature babies who weigh less than one and a half pounds and are unlikely to survive	7	9	10	10
Long stay care	8	10	3	6
Community services or care at home	9	5	1	3
Health education services (campaigns encouraging healthy lifestyles)	10	8	8	8
Treatments for infertility	11	11	11	11

Sources: Ham,[10] Bowling,[11], OPCS Omnibus May–June 1995. Adapted from ranking exercises that involved up to 16 services. For means of comparison, only those services that appeared in *both* the 1992 and 1995 surveys are retained.

Table 5.4 Priority rating of specific health service: public and expert opinion

Services or treatments	Public, MORI (1993): $n = 2012$	Public, Gallup (Aug. 1994): $n = 1027$	Doctors (1993): $n = 761$	Managers (1993): $n = 266$
Childhood immunisation	1	2	1	1
Screening for breast cancer	2	3	7	5
Care offered by GPs	3	1	2	2 =
Intensive care for premature babies	4	5	8	8
Heart transplants	5	7	9 =	9
Support for carers of elderly people	6	4	3 =	4
Hip replacement for elderly people	7	8	5	6
Education to prevent young people smoking	8	6	3 =	2 =
Treatment for schizophrenia	9	10	6	7
Cancer treatment for smokers	10	9	9 =	10

Sources: Heginbotham,[7] MORI 1993; Gallup 9.8.94–15.8.94

Table 5.5 Priority rating of specific health services: public and expert opinion

Treatments	Forum participants, Mid-Essex: $n = 13$	Public health directors, Mid-Essex: $n = 68$
Breast screening	1	6
Cataract removal	2	2
Hip replacement	3	1
Renal dialysis	4	4
Heart bypass	5	3
Treatment for AIDS	6	7
Neonatal care	7	8
Hernias	8	5
Treatment for advanced Parkinson's disease	9	9
Liver transplantations	10	11
Treatment for advanced lung cancer	11	12
Heart transplantations	12	10

Source: Lutton and Carroll.[13]

Table 5.6 Prioritising types of treatments

Year	Methodology	Statement	Agree (Disagree) (%)	Don't know (%)
1994 (Aug)	National survey, Gallup: $n = 1027$	Funds should be concentrated on those treatments that improve the quality of many people's lives	87 7	7
1995	National survey, OPCS Omnibus $n = 1975$	The patient's quality of life should be considered in determining whether or not to use lifesaving treatment/technology	74 14	12
1993	National survey, MORI: $n = 2012$	Choose between: Treatment that greatly improves people's ability to lead a normal life but is not life threatening ...	57	13
		or treatment that saves people's lives but often means that they are unable to lead a normal life	31	
1992	Local survey City and Hackney: $n = 335$	Preventing illness is at least as important as curing it	77 13	10
		It is more important to treat people who are ill than it is to prevent illness	36 41	23

Sources: Gallup 9.8.94–15.8.94; Bowling,[11] OPCS Omnibus May–June 1995; Heginbotham,[7] MORI 1993; Bowling.[14]

between 77% and 81% of the respondents rated cancer care for the dying, neonatal intensive care, childhood immunisation, and screening services as "essential", with cosmetic surgery and fertility services regarded as the two most "unimportant" services provided by the NHS.[12]

We can also see from Tables 5.3 and 5.4 that the priority rankings of the public were reasonably close to the professionals'. In Table 5.3, both the public and expert opinion rated treatments for children with life

Table 5.7   Prioritising types of treatments (row percentages)

Priority (rank)	1 (most important)	2 %	3 %	4 %	5 (least important)
Health care that **prolongs the life and reduces** pain or disability in people who are severely ill or disabled	36	31	15	14	4
Health care that **prevents** illness among people who are currently well	38	20	19	16	7
Health care that **improves** mental health in people who are severely mentally ill	13	19	32	26	10
Health care that does **not prolong life but does reduce** pain or disability in people who are severely ill	13	24	24	23	16
Health care that prolongs life but **does not reduce** pain or disability in people who are severely ill or disabled	2	7	10	19	62

Sources: Bowling;[14] City and Hackney local survey, N = 335.

threatening illnesses highly and treatments for infertility at the bottom. Significant differences in opinion were, however, also detected. First, the public would appear to rank high technology surgery (such as a heart transplantation) more highly than the professionals. Second, the public appears to view mental health care, long stay care, and community care as lower priorities than the doctors and managers. These findings are replicated in Table 5.4. There, differences in public and expert opinion existed over the relative importance of heart transplantations, treatment for schizophrenia, screening for breast cancer, intensive care for pre-term babies, and education to prevent young people smoking.

That said, where there were differences in the public and professional view, it can be argued that public opinion is moving towards the experts' standpoint. In Table 5.3, the public ranking of high technology surgery is considerably closer to the expert view in the later of the two polls. The same can be said of the public's view on community services. In Table 5.4, a similar trend is evident. On each of the ranking of heart transplantations, support for carers, and education to prevent young people smoking, the more recent of the public surveys shows the public's view moving closer to professional opinion. Indeed, in the nine cases (in either table) of public opinion on a treatment's priority changing by two or more ranks, the public view moves towards expert opinion seven times. Only once does it move in the opposite direction (long stay care, Table 5.3).

Table 5.5 offers another example of public and professional rankings of specific services or treatments. However, in contrast to Tables 5.3 and 5.4,

67

the evidence is from a more deliberative form of polling: a public health forum.

The first notable difference between Table 5.5 and Tables 5.3 and 5.4 is the fact that the public view (forum participants) is very similar to that of the professionals (public health directors). The only real differences are over the position of breast screening (again ranked more highly by the public) and hernia operations (ranked more highly by the directors). This form of deliberative polling, where the public can talk decisions through, appears to bring public opinion closer to that of expert opinion. Opinion on the position of hip replacements, neonatal care, and heart transplantations are consistent between lay and professional views. This form of considered decision making may counter the effects of a lack of information which has been recognised as one cause of the public's lack of consistency in opinion poll surveys.[7] More evidence from this type of methodology is required, however, before we can be sure.

Other measures of public opinion on treatment priorities elicit from the public a more *general* opinion (Tables 5.6 and 5.7). It seems that, despite prioritising high technology life saving treatments (especially for children), the public places treatment that preserves quality of life above life saving interventions (MORI 1993). It is also clear from Table 5.6 that preventing illness is seen to be at least as important as curing it (77% agreement, City and Hackney survey 1992). It may even be perceived to be more important (41% agreement, City and Hackney survey 1992).

Evidence from Table 5.7 supports these general views. In the City and Hackney survey, respondents preferred treatments that reduced pain, prevented illness, or improved health to that which prolonged life but did not reduce suffering. However, it should be noticed that these *general* views are not entirely consistent with the *specific* rankings of Tables 5.3 and 5.4 where intensive care for pre-term babies and treatments for children with life threatening illnesses (both interventionist measures) were ranked higher than mental health care and education to prevent young people smoking. It may be that the public answers the general questions less emotionally than it does the specific ones. If this is the case, the two categories of opinion should be analysed together by policy makers in order to come to a considered view.[7]

What patient groups are priorities?

Which patients, as well as services or treatments, should have a high priority is another theme on which public views have been elicited. As before, most of the available evidence is based on survey data. However, as with the last section, some evidence from decisions taken in focus groups is available to us.

Table 5.8   Public views on prioritising patients

Year	Methodology	Statement	Agree (Disagree) (%)	Don't know (%)
1995	National survey, OPCS Omnibus: n = 1975	If resources must be rationed, higher priority should be given to treating young than elderly	50 29	21
		High cost technology . . . should be available to all regardless of age	80 13	7
1994 (Aug)	National survey, Gallup: n = 1027	If people are very old and very ill, their lives should not be prolonged by expensive treatment	31 52	16
		Here are some groups of people. Which of them, in your view, should have priority for receiving health care?:		
		Previously healthy young and middle aged people	16	
		People with family responsibilities?	28	
		Small babies?	26	
		The mentally ill?	3	
		The terminally ill?	6	
		Retired people?	3	
		People with self-inflicted illnesses or injuries?	0	
		None/all equal?	3	
		Don't know		30

Sources: Bowling 1996,[11] OPCS Omnibus May–June 1995; Gallup 9.8.94–15.8.94.

The main thrust of the question of prioritising patient groups deals with the perceived need to give *high priority* to some categories of people and *low priority* to others in the provision of health care. In terms of high priority, the choice is often seen to be between young and old people. In terms of low priority, however, the question most often asked of the public is whether those people who bring their illnesses on themselves, or at least contribute to their illnesses, deserve to be prioritised as highly as those who do not.

On the first question, it is clear from Table 5.8 that the public is not consistent in its views. Although 50% of the respondents in the OPCS Omnibus survey agreed that "higher priority should be given to treating the young than the elderly", 80% agreed that "high cost technology . . . should be available to all regardless of age". In the Gallup survey, moreover, 52% disagreed with the statement, "if people are very old and very ill, their lives should not be prolonged by expensive treatment". That said, when the same respondents were asked to prioritise *groups* of people, public opinion appeared to switch back to prioritising the young. Top priority for healthcare treatment was accorded to "people with family responsibilities", "small babies", and "previously healthy young and middle-aged people".

Table 5.9   Public views on prioritising patients

Year	Methodology	Statement	Agree (Disagree) (%)	Don't know (%)
1994 (Aug)	National survey, Gallup: n = 1027	People who bring their illnesses on themselves—by, for example, smoking or drinking heavily—should be lower down the queue for NHS care than other patients	41 49	10
1995	National survey, OPCS Omnibus n = 1975	People who contribute to their own illness . . . should have lower priority for their health care than others	42 43	15
1994 (Jun)	National survey, Gallup: n = 989	Which of the following types of people, if any, do you think should go to the back of the queue for hospital treatment:		
		Smokers?	25 (67)	7
		Overweight?	11 (82)	7
		Heavy drinkers?	32 (60)	8
		People who overwork?	7 (86)	7
1995	Focus group, Somerset	Should coronary bypass operations be denied to all smokers altogether?	1 99	0
		Should coronary bypass operations be denied to smokers who refuse to give up smoking?	25 75	0
		Should smokers have low priority for coronary bypass operations, compared to other people?	28 72	0

Sources: Bowling,[11] OPCS Omnibus May–June 1995; Gallup 9.8.94–15.8.94; Gallup June 1994; Bowie et al.[15].

The group entitled "retired people" were felt to be the top priority for health care by only 3% of the respondents.

This inconsistency of opinion is magnified by the fact that for the four questions listed in Table 5.8, the average number of "don't knows" is 18·5%. One respondent in five generally failed to either agree or disagree with a statement or to choose a group for prioritising. It may be, however, that, as with the question on the necessity of rationing, changes in question wording are crucial. For instance, when the public is presented with a direct choice between young and old people, young people are always prioritised (OPCS Omnibus 1995 and Gallup 1994). This is consistent with the earlier findings that saw the public rate treatments for children with life threatening illnesses higher than other life saving interventions such as heart transplantations (Table 5.3).

The evidence that deals with *relegating* groups of patients to a lower priority is seemingly less volatile. Of the two questions in Table 5.9 which ask about the priority to be accorded to those people who bring illness on themselves (Gallup August 1994 and OPCS Omnibus 1995), the public is almost evenly split on each occasion. Both measures show that the public is opposed—by a small majority—to relegating such groups of patients. However, when the question posed is more *specific* (that is, should smokers be given lower priority?), opposition to relegating these specific groups of patients is increased. For example, in the June 1994 Gallup poll, only 25% of the respondents favoured pushing smokers to the back of the queue. Corresponding figures of 11%, 32%, and 7% were recorded for the "overweight", "heavy drinkers", and "people who overwork" respectively.

Similar opinions were apparent in the evidence from the focus groups conducted in Somerset and Bromley. In Somerset, the questions posed were more complex and the decisions arrived at were more considered. Moreover, it seems that this measure of public opinion was more consensual in its decision. First, it was agreed by 99% of the public polled that heart bypass operations should not be denied to smokers altogether. Second, 75% of the respondents believed that bypass operations should not be denied to smokers who refuse to give up. And third, 72% disagreed with the notion that smokers should "have low priority for coronary bypass operations, compared to other people". This broad agreement was replicated by other decisions taken by community groups and citizens' juries.[17] As with the evidence from the Mid-Essex Public Health Forum in the last section, however, to be certain about the validity of these findings, more research is needed on these particular methodologies.

Who should make the decisions?

If the public accepts that the NHS *does* have to prioritise types of treatments and groups of patients, they would appear to have a clear view on who should make the decisions. In short, decisions should be left to the "experts"—in most cases doctors—with Health Service managers, the Government and, importantly for this analysis, the general public having an input in the decision making process.

All the available evidence would seem to concur with this view. With respect to Tables 5.10 and 5.11, it seems that, although the public does not want to *make* the decisions over what to prioritise, they feel that they should be *part of the process* of reaching a decision. Poll after poll—at the local level, the national level, and in group decision making—shows a similar message.

In Table 5.10, for instance, 75% of the respondents in the OPCS Omnibus poll agreed that doctors should decide on priorities. For the Gallup poll this figure is 61%. The corresponding figures at the local level, where the question asked was again slightly different, are 58% and 59%, respectively. Even allowing for variations in question wording, the public's view seems unambiguous: doctors—not managers, politicians, or the general public—should be left with the *final* decision over what to prioritise.

Table 5.10   Public views on decision-making

Year	Methodology	Statement	Agree (Disagree) (%)	Don't know (%)
1995	National survey, OPCS Omnibus: $n = 1975$	The responsibility to ration health care spending should rest with the doctor rather than a hospital manager, health authority, politician, or government minister	75 15	10
1994 (Aug)	National survey, Gallup: $n = 1027$	To the extent that the NHS has to establish priorities, who do you think should do it ... (Some respondents chose more than one group)		
		Health Service managers?	14	
		Doctors?	61	
		Government?	9	
		General public?	17	
		Other?	1	
		Don't know.		7
		Should decisions in these matters be left mainly to the [group(s) mentioned above] ...	49	10
		or should the general public ... have a large say in the matter	42	
1990	Local survey, Bath: $n = 690$	Decisions should be left to the doctors and other experts at the health authority	58 39	3
1992	Local survey, City and Hackney: $n = 213$	Decisions should be left to the doctors and other experts at the health authority	59 21	20

Sources: Bowling,[11] Omnibus May–June 1995; Gallup 9.8.94–15.8.94; Bowling;[14] Richardson et al.[17]

Significantly, this consistency of opinion is replicated when the public comes to consider its own role in the decision making process. In the Gallup poll (Table 5.10), 42% of the respondents felt that the public should have "a large say" in the matter of prioritising. In the Bath and City and Hackney surveys (Table 5.11), where the corresponding phrase reads "more of a say" in making decisions, agreement with the notion of public consultation rises to 65% and 67%, respectively. This trend is supported by evidence from elsewhere. In the OPCS Omnibus survey, 88% of the respondents believed that "surveys of the general public's opinions, such as this one, should be used in the planning of health services".[11] Finally, as we would expect from the evidence put forward in the previous sections, at the Cambridge and Huntingdon citizens' jury the decision was even more consensual. There, it was agreed by a majority of 15–1 that "there should be an element of public involvement in developing guidelines for priority setting".[16]

Table 5.11 What role should the public play?

Year	Methodology	Statement	Agree (Disagree) (%)	Don't know (%)
1990	Local survey, Bath: n = 690	The public should have more of a say in making the decisions (on priority setting)	65 27	7
1992	Local survey, City and Hackney: n = 213	The public should have more of a say in making the decisions (on priority setting)	67 13	20
1995	National survey, OPCS Omnibus: n = 1975	Surveys of the general public's opinions, such as this one, should be used in the planning of health services	88 7	5
1996	Citizens' jury, Cambridge and Huntingdon	The public should be involved in developing guidelines for priority setting	94 6	0

Sources: Richardson et al.[17]; Bowling[11,14]; OPCS Omnibus May-June 1995; Lenaghan[16].

The evidence is both overwhelming and at odds with the view that the public generally wishes to defer authority in healthcare priority setting to doctors and other "experts".[18] What is more, the evidence serves to counteract the impression—given by poor turnouts at public meetings[19]—that the public does not want to be involved in priority setting. The reverse is actually true. The message, at least so far as we can see, is that although the final decision on priorities should be left with doctors, the public is willing to contribute in the development of guidelines in health service priority setting.

Discussion: understanding the differences in public opinion

Aside from simply reporting on the state of public opinion and health care rationing, one of the themes of this chapter has been the separation of evidence from mass opinion polls and the more focused methodologies. We have seen from the small number of data in our possession that, when the public is exposed to information, its views seem to move closer to those expressed by "experts" (Table 5.4). At the same time we have seen that decisions taken in a group context have been more consensual (Tables 5.9 and 5.11). What, then, are we to make of these apparent differences of public opinion?

Surveys/opinion polls	Public meetings	Health forums Community groups	Focus groups	Citizens' juries

Exposure to health care information ➡
Correlation with the views of "experts" ➡
Degree of consensus of decision ➡

Fig. 5.1 Different measures of public opinion according to information exposure

Are all measures of public opinion the same?

Analysis of public opinion on health care is disadvantaged by the fact that, for the most part, the public remains ignorant of the detail of healthcare planning. It is clear from the last three sections, however, that the public questioned in surveys do not hold exactly the same views as those members of the public who take part in focus groups and citizens' juries. At the heart of this difference is the varying level of information to which individual members of the public are exposed. In the case of survey respondents, the level of information to which the individual is exposed is virtually nil. When public views are elicited from focus groups and citizens' juries, however, these views are the product of greater information. Along these lines, one commentator has observed that "it may be that some of the difference in ranking between the public and doctors and managers is because doctors and managers have far more knowledge about the costs and benefits of different treatments".[7] This would seem to be the case. When the public *does* become more knowledgeable their opinions converge on those held by healthcare professionals (Fig. 5.1).

Nevertheless, we need more evidence from these deliberative methodologies to be certain of our conclusions. Until we can measure public opinion from focus groups and citizens' juries, and compare it with survey data on a wider basis, our hypothesis that information exposure influences public opinion remains just that: a hypothesis. It does seem to be a realistic one, however, and worthy of closer examination. Certainly, blaming the public for its own lack of information is not an option:[7]

> The public responds to information made available. If that information is insufficient then the problem of providing more information should be addressed by health authorities, managers, and clinicians.

(pp 152–3)

Conclusion

What, if anything, does this mean for public opinion and health care rationing? To begin with, it seems clear that informing the public is crucial

74

if public opinion is to be used in the process of priority setting. Put simply, it would seem to be more defensible for policy makers (or anybody else interested in public opinion) to elicit *informed* rather than *uninformed* public views on health care. Second, the quality of our understanding about public opinion and health care would be considerably improved if there were a focused effort to collect comparable information on a routine basis over time. This is essential if we are to distinguish between fluctuations in public opinion and the vagaries of specific methods of data collection.

Third, it is clear, however, that the public can learn. It can appreciate the dilemmas implicit in the allocation of health care resources and it can respond intelligently to the evidence that is presented to it. For the Rationing Agenda Group, this is probably the most important, and heartening, finding.

Summary

(1) **A number of different methods have been used to elicit public opinion on healthcare rationing.** These range from undertaking surveys, both local and national, to analysing the decisions taken, or views expressed, by community groups, focus groups, citizens' juries and public meetings. The most common method is the use of surveys.

(2) **On the question of the necessity of rationing, it is not clear what the public thinks.** The evidence that we have seems to be contradictory. The main problem is that most of the evidence we possess comes from survey data that are not strictly comparable due to differences in question wording.

(3) **In terms of prioritising *specific services or treatments*, significant differences were detected between public and professional opinion.** The public appear to rate high technology surgery and screening for breast cancer more highly than the professionals but mental health care, long stay care and community care lower than the professionals. These differences were less clear when public opinion was elicited via a health forum where the public's views were the product of considered opinion. When asked *general* policy questions, however, it seems the public places treatment that preserves quality of life above life saving interventions. This is in line with professional opinion.

(4) **In terms of *prioritising patients*, the public's view is uncertain.** Some evidence suggests that the young should be prioritised at the expense of the old whilst some suggests that age should make no difference to the provision of health care. When asked to make a direct choice between young and old, however, the young are always prioritised. With regard to people who contribute to their own illness, when *specific* groups (e.g. smokers) are mentioned, most people feel that they should *not* be relegated to the back of the queue for health care.

(5) When it comes to deciding who should make the decisions over what to prioritise, the public's view is unambiguous: **decisions should be left to doctors, with health service managers, the government and the**

general public involved in the process. That is, though the public does not want to *make* the decisions over what to prioritise, it is clear that they feel that their views should be taken into account.

(6) **All analyses of public opinion on health care are disadvantaged by the fact that, for the most part, the public remains relatively ignorant of detail.**

(7) **All public opinion is not the same.** When the public is exposed to information about health care—in citizens' juries for example—its views change in two ways. First, the public's views move closer to those expressed by doctors and managers. Second, public opinion becomes more consensual.

(8) **Informing the public is crucial if public opinion is to be used in the process of priority setting.** It would seem to be more defensible to elicit *informed* rather than *uninformed* public views.

1 Department of Health. *The Patient's Charter.* London: HMSO, 1992.
2 National Health Service Management Executive. *Local voices: the views of local people in purchasing for health.* London: Department of Health, 1992.
3 Bowling A, Jacobson B, Southgate L. Health service priorities: explorations in consultation of the public and health professionals on priority setting in an inner London health district. *Soc Sci Med* 1993;37:851–7.
4 McIver S. Information for public choice. *Br Med Bull* 1995;51:900–13.
5 Donovan J, Coast J. Public preferences in priority setting: unresolved issues. In Malek, M. (ed.) *Setting priorities in health care.* Chichester: John Wiley & Sons, 1994;32.
6 Jacobson B, Bowling A. Involving the public: practical and ethical issues. *Br Med Bull* 1995;51:869–75.
7 Heginbotham C. Health care priority setting: a survey of doctors, managers, and the general public. In Smith R. (ed.), *Rationing in action.* London: BMJ Publishing, 1993.
8 Dicker A, Armstrong, D. Patients' views of priority setting in health care: an interview survey on one practice. *BMJ* 1995;311:1137–9.
9 Barker J. *Local NHS health care purchasing and prioritising from the perspective of Bromley residents—a qualitative study.* Bromley Health: Hayes, 1995.
10 Ham C. Priority setting in the NHS: reports from six districts. *BMJ* 1993;307:435–8.
11 Bowling A. Health care rationing: the public's debate. *BMJ* 1996;312:670–4.
12 MacDonald LD. *Determining community priorities in health care: report to East Surrey Health Authority.* University of London, 1992.
13 Lutton G, Carroll G. *Fourth public health forum.* Mid-Essex Health Authority, 1991.
14 Bowling A. *What people say about prioritising health services.* London: King's Fund Centre, 1993.
15 Bowie C, Richardson A, Sykes W. Consulting the public about health service priorities. *BMJ* 1995;311:1155–8.
16 Lenaghan J, New B, Mitchell E. Setting priorities: is there a role for citizens' juries? *BMJ* 1996;312:1591–3.
17 Richardson A, Charny M, Hanmer-Lloyd S. Public opinion and purchasing. *BMJ* 1992; 304:680–2.
18 Klein R, Day P, Redmayne S. *Managing scarcity: priority setting and rationing in the National Health Service.* Buckingham: Open University Press, 1996.
19 Timmins N. How would *you* spend the health service budget? *Independent* 12/3/93.

The rationing debate

As part of its mission to raise the level of debate about rationing of healthcare resources, the Rationing Agenda Group commissioned six pairs of articles debating specific propositions to do with rationing. These articles are all contained within this section, including some extra rejoinders.

6 Defining a package of healthcare services the NHS is responsible for

There is a need for a clearly defined package of healthcare services which is relevant to, and the responsibility of, the NHS

The case for

BILL NEW

The use of tattoo removal as an example of NHS rationing is now so common that it is in danger of trivialising an important debate. Behind such questions as "Should the NHS be devoting resources to tattoo removal?" lies a more fundamental issue: what *kinds* of benefit should the NHS provide?

Most readers will assume that defining a healthcare "package" is a means of rationing healthcare resources. In other words, faced with the task of managing the limited NHS budget one option is to exclude some services altogether. But my case rests on a different interpretation of a package and involves asking a preliminary question. Before deciding how to ration, we need to know what to ration: What is the range of services relevant to the role of the NHS? What "business" is the NHS in? Is it the NHS's job to provide fertility treatment, physiotherapy for sports injuries, long term nursing care, sex reassignment, adult dentistry, and cosmetic surgery? Or should these services be provided by local authorities, voluntary agencies, or the private sector? The question does not rely on clinical judgment. It is about the boundary of a public institution's responsibilities. And it is a question that has been muddled up with issues of rationing proper.

Defining the boundaries

The need to address this question derives from a growing sense of confusion and uncertainty about what it is reasonable to expect from the

NHS. For example, where one lives can have a decisive effect on whether or not NHS treatment is available. The 1991 NHS reforms were an important catalyst in this process: purchasing authorities now concentrate on commissioning health care for their resident populations, rather than on management issues. Wishing to be seen to be making the best use of financial allocations, some took the view that certain services were not a priority and therefore not worth purchasing. For example, the availability of fertility treatment depends on the whim of purchasing health authorities—and increasingly general practice fundholders. In addition to this uncertainty over regional variations is the apparent removal of some primary care services from NHS provision altogether. Adult dentistry is subsidised by central government, but only for a fraction of its cost. In some areas it is hard to find dentists who offer even this minimal NHS cover. There has been no explicit national debate about why dentistry is apparently not an NHS responsibility.

It is inequitable that one's place of residence should determine access to care. Levels of service provision will inevitably vary from one part of the country to another, in response to varying need or because some providers are more efficient than others. But this is different from removing availability altogether: infertility is not at zero levels in those areas where in vitro fertilisation treatment it is not available. Ad hoc developments such as these can serve only to promote uncertainty and a sense of unfairness quite out of proportion to the quantity of resources at stake. Furthermore, the vigilance of the news media has had a significant impact on the public's perception of health delivery. Activity, and inactivity, in the NHS are now scrutinised and reported daily. This is welcome, but awkward: old issues, once hidden, must now be tackled if the NHS is not to fall into disrepute.

Nothing to do with saving money

To be clear about what devising a healthcare package would seek to achieve, we must be clear about what it is not trying to do. First, it is not (necessarily) about saving money. The case for a centrally defined package has been associated with easing the pressure on resources. However, this is not the purpose of the proposals outlined here—the desire is to promote equity, collective understanding, and reassurance. The package considered relevant to NHS business is just as likely to be more extensive than that available now. The point is that it should not vary from one area to another and that it should be derived as the result of an explicit, democratic process.

Second, drawing up such a package is not an attempt to avoid additional rationing. In the well-known Oregon initiative in the USA, all those services that might possibly be provided collectively are ranked and the line drawn where resources allow. Above the line everyone has access; below no one does (unless privately financed). The line moves up and down depending on the availability of resources. Rationing health care is therefore a centrally undertaken activity, specifying a package to which everyone has access.

But the approach presented here is a preliminary to rationing. It is about deciding what should appear on Oregon's list in total, not about where the line should be drawn. Of course, there will be resource implications from this decision. For example, if long term nursing care was considered an NHS responsibility then resources might need to be reallocated from private households to the NHS through taxation. But specifying a package to promote reassurance and geographical fairness does not involve deciding how NHS resources should be distributed between individuals who make a claim on them. Defining a package does not imply a right to treatment.

Cost effectiveness not relevant to establishing "the package"

If the need, in principle, for a package is accepted, however, then there must be a coherent and practical means of establishing it. For this to be successful the focus must shift from criteria that guide rationing decisions to criteria that help establish the range of relevant services which are to be rationed. Trying to do both at once results in doing very little at all, as international experience testifies.

New Zealand and the Netherlands have both tried to establish packages of healthcare services, and both have had little success. In New Zealand, "core" services were intended both to clarify what the population could expect and limit the financial burden on the state. Ultimately, though, the planners were forced to concede that everything that was currently provided would form the core—hardly the result they were looking for. In the Netherlands, four criteria—necessity, effectiveness, efficiency, and individual responsibility—were used to define a package. The Dutch also found it difficult to specify precisely which services ought to be excluded. Why so little success?

These strategies were trying to do too much at once. Issues of equity, reassurance, and clarity about the responsibility of the state were mixed up with a desire to contain costs and ration more systematically. The root of the difficulties lies in the inclusion of effectiveness and cost effectiveness as criteria for establishing a package.

Whether a service is relevant to a healthcare system has nothing to do with effectiveness. For example, cosmetic surgery for enhancement where there is no severe psychological distress is rarely supported for collective healthcare provision. But no one suggests that the plastic surgeons who work miracles on Hollywood stars are not effective. So questions of

81

effectiveness and cost effectiveness should be left aside at this stage of the debate.

Their importance comes when deciding how to allocate resources between all the services that are relevant and between the people who can benefit from them. The result of such deliberations may also lead to a package, but it will be of an entirely different kind. In Oregon, cost effectiveness was the basic principle at work (although with many refinements and alongside other criteria). But the resulting package did not address whether fertility treatment, residential care, dentistry, and so on were relevant to Oregon's public healthcare provision.

Reliance on measures of cost and effectiveness has meant that most commentators believe strategies for defining a package are doomed to failure, or at least likely to disappoint those who promote them.[1] The reasons given are now reasonably well accepted: health interventions are extremely variable in their effects on individuals. Just about every treatment therefore does some good for someone, even if it is "ineffective" in general. Making blanket exclusions on this basis will inevitably be a blunt instrument and will antagonise doctors, who feel their clinical freedom is curtailed. As a consequence, the Oregon experiment has proved to be extremely controversial and has generally not been considered relevant to the NHS.

A qualitative approach

But the following approach for establishing relevance to the NHS does not rely on effectiveness. Instead it proposes a qualitative approach which avoids the difficulties of variable individual response to treatment. The approach has been described in more detail elsewhere,[2] but the central proposition is this: those characteristics which define healthcare's special nature, and which in general terms make it unsuitable for economic exchange, should determine whether or not individual services are relevant to the NHS.

Taken together, three characteristics set health care apart: fundamental importance, information imbalance, and uncertainty. Health is clearly of fundamental importance; there is little certainty about how our health will develop in the future; and typically we know little about the nature of our needs for health care or of the likely effects of the treatments available to us. In short, we are not good consumers. We must trust doctors who, under free market conditions with insurance markets, have an incentive to provide as much care as possible.

It is the combination of characteristics which makes health care special. Fundamental importance is not sufficient on its own—food, after all, is important but no one suggests that we should have a National Food Service because people are perfectly able to choose what and how much food they need. Neither are information imbalance and uncertainty sufficient on their own. Car repair services display these characteristics, but no one is suggesting a National Car Repair Service—because cars are not of fundamental importance.

However, not all services which are related to health care display these characteristics in combination. Residential care for elderly people is fundamentally important but does not suffer from significant information imbalances; cosmetic surgery for enhancement is not generally considered to be of fundamental importance. Services of this kind should not be an NHS responsibility. On the other hand, curative dentistry, fertility treatment, and intensive nursing care do seem to satisfy the criteria; consequently, they should form part of the NHS's range of available services. All health authorities and GP fundholders should be required to provide some level of these services. Note that defining this package does not imply any judgment about effectiveness or whether any individual service represents good value for money. It simply clarifies what the NHS should be in the business of doing.

Meeting the objections

There are a several practical objections to such a proposal. The first argues that such an approach necessitates drawing up a long list of individual services which would need to be continually updated. Every existing and new treatment for cancer for example, would need specification. In fact, such an enterprise would be unnecessary. Specification is required only at a general level: treatment for cancer, AIDS, infertility, or whatever, not individual drugs or surgical interventions. Indeed, it may be sufficient simply to concentrate on exclusions rather than long lists of inclusions. Furthermore, whether or not a particular treatment is effective is irrelevant—the NHS may decide not to purchase a drug to treat AIDS until it proves its effectiveness, but it would be clear that drugs of this kind are relevant to NHS business.

The second objection argues that any attempt to centralise decision making will fail to accommodate individual cases and exceptional circumstances. Clearly, defining the range of relevant services will restrict clinicians' ability to use their skills to certain ends. But this will not be as inflexible as critics suggest.

A typical example cites an individual with extreme psychological distress caused by a tattoo mistakenly purchased when young. In circumstances where cosmetic surgery for enhancement is outside NHS responsibilities, surely such central codification would deny legitimate treatment? Not if treatment is correctly focused on the nature of the condition. In the case of psychological distress the correct course of action is referral to a psychiatrist (psychiatry, let us assume, is within NHS responsibilities). The specialist might well provide appropriate treatment herself or may recommend removal of the tattoo as the preferred means of treating the distress. In this way tattoo removal could still be undertaken quite legitimately on the NHS. But at the same time some restriction has been placed on clinical freedom: cosmetic procedures for conditions that do not involve psychological distress are outside the scope of the NHS—no exceptions. If a real improvement in the clarity of the NHS's role and equity in the availability of its services is to be achieved then such restrictions are inevitable.

The final objection asserts that introducing legal specifications of what the NHS should provide will simply allow the nominal provision of services. So, for example, if infertility were to be included it would probably be sufficient for a health authority to provide one round of treatment per year to satisfy its legal obligations. Thus health authorities could pay lip service to the policy but continue to decide the range of responsibilities for themselves. This may indeed turn out to be how purchasers act. But it is equally reasonable to suppose that health authorities simply want clear guidance on the range of their responsibilities and have no wish to indulge in gamesmanship with policy directives. In any event, individual purchasers would be clear about their role—they would still decide on the extent of provision depending on local circumstances, but would now provide services secure in the knowledge that they were in step with all other purchasers in the NHS.

One final point. Criteria such as those suggested here for guiding the specification of a healthcare package are just that: guidance. They cannot replace debate and political compromise. So it is not possible simply to read off a list of relevant healthcare services—people will inevitably disagree over the degree to which fertility treatment, for example, satisfies information imbalance and fundamental importance. But once a decision has been made, openly and with reference to coherent criteria, what we stand to gain from clarity and equity will surely outweigh the awkward processes involved. The alternative—allowing the NHS increasingly to ignore the principles on which it was founded—risks losing mass popular respect for a successful and valued public institution.

1 Klein R. Can we restrict the health care menu? *Health Policy* 1994;27:103–12.
2 New B, Le Grand J. *Rationing in the NHS: principles and pragmatism.* London: King's Fund, 1996.

The case against

RUDOLF KLEIN

Traditionally the National Health Service has relied on implicit rationing by clinicians within budgetary constraints set by central government. Neither the founding fathers, nor any of their successors, defined the scope and limits of the NHS's responsibilities. The statutory responsibility of ministers of health is to provide an "adequate" service. But the frontiers of adequacy have never been defined, and the courts have resolutely refused to rule on what should be provided to whom. The package of health care offered has thus varied, in terms of its composition and its generosity, both over time and geographically. It is for individual health authorities to decide what package of healthcare services to provide for their populations and for individual clinicians to decide between the competing claims on the resources available to them.[1]

Unsatisfactory state of affairs

In many ways this is an unsatisfactory state of affairs and not surprisingly has increasingly come under challenge. There are two main grounds for criticism. First, the present situation allows ministers to duck responsibility for the consequences of their decisions when setting the NHS's budget. If "adequacy" remains an elastic and fuzzy notion, there is no way of establishing whether the budget is sufficient to meet the NHS's commitments. Without any definition of what those commitments are in the first place, the debate about whether or not the NHS is "underfunded" becomes a meaningless dialogue of the deaf and accountability is fudged. Second, the lack of any defined package means that in practice there can be no equity, if by equity is meant that everyone should have the same opportunity of treatment for any given degree of need for a particular healthcare intervention. A considerable degree of arbitrariness remains in the chances of getting treated in the NHS: even if equity were achieved in terms of ensuring that all health authorities have the same command over resources, relative to the needs of their populations, there would still be no assurance that they would necessarily buy the same set of services. Developments since the introduction of the 1991 NHS reforms have reinforced these general considerations. The medical profession has become increasingly restive about having to carry the ultimate responsibility for rationing. If resources are short, many doctors now argue, ministers should accept the burden of determining what can or cannot be provided. Further, the purchaser-provider split has given visibility to decisions by health authorities about what care to buy—or not to buy—for their populations. The visibility may be less than complete, but enough has been revealed to cause disquiet about the differences of policy that have emerged. For example, it would seem absurd that the chances of getting in vitro fertilisation treatment should depend on where people live, yet health authorities differ sharply on whether or not to buy this treatment.[2]

The case for defining the package of healthcare services to be delivered by the NHS is therefore strong. I will argue, however, that the case against moving in this direction is even stronger—for four main reasons. First, no consensus exists about the principles or criteria that should be used in designing such a package. Second, any decisions to restrict the NHS menu are difficult to implement, given patient heterogeneity. Third, by concentrating on rationing by denial we risk ignoring other (probably more important) dimensions of rationing. Fourth, defining an NHS package would probably not achieve the declared objectives of promoting equity and accountability, and the all out pursuit of these objectives would in any case lead to a damaging degree of centralised rigidity.

A perplexity of criteria

The case for defining the NHS menu assumes the feasibility of developing criteria acceptable to both public and professionals for determining what should be included and excluded. And indeed many such criteria are on offer. The growing international interest in limiting the open ended financial commitments of healthcare systems has, in turn, produced a series of attempts to develop principles for defining the limits of national packages. The result of all this activity is, however, discouraging. A cacophony of criteria is on offer, embodying competing (and sometimes conflicting) views about how to define the limits of public responsibility for health care. And when seemingly uncontentious criteria are proposed, it turns out that their acceptability depends crucially on their level of abstraction: acceptable as general propositions, they become contentious when applied to particular cases.

International experience

The problem of conflicting criteria is well illustrated by the international experience.[1] Oregon's much cited exercise in defining a package of care for those not covered by medical insurance was originally based on ranking different conditions–treatments according to their cost–benefit ratio. It thus embodied the economist's notion that any package of care should be designed to maximise the community's return on any resources invested in health care. In the outcome this was effectively abandoned, partly because adequate data were lacking, partly because the exercise produced some counterintuitive results—for example, appendectomy ranked lower than tooth capping. The final rankings that appeared, after repeated massaging, seem to reflect judgments about "reasonableness" taken in the light of community values. In other words, the attempt to apply clear cut, transparent criteria was abandoned.

The Dunning committee, which sought to develop criteria for defining a package of health care for the Netherlands, proposed four criteria for including any intervention or services: necessity, effectiveness, efficiency, and whether it is a matter of individual, rather than community, responsibility. Necessary services were those that "guarantee normal functions as a member of the community or simply protect existence as a member". It thus recognised both economic considerations and the "rule of rescue"—that conditions that threaten survival or the capacity to function must be included in any package. So, for example, in vitro fertilisation failed to pass the necessity test: "Undesired childlessness in the Netherlands poses no danger to the community, and it cannot be said that childlessness interferes with normal function in our society."

In contrast, a Swedish commission rejected outright the efficiency principle—that is, the economistic approach to defining a basic package. Instead, it endorsed the rule of rescue by giving priority to the treatment of life threatening conditions. It also invoked social solidarity—the principle that the commitments of a healthcare system should be shaped by a sense of collective responsibility for the wellbeing of its members, especially the most vulnerable, such as chronically and terminally ill individuals. And the New Zealand committee on core services declined the task of defining the contents or limits of a healthcare package.

Defining characteristics of health care

The list of possible criteria could be extended further. Consider, for example, a recent, highly ingenious attempt to cut through the confusion by deriving the principles for defining the basic package from the arguments used to justify public intervention in the provision of health care in the first place. Public provision or financing is justified, New and Le Grand argue,[3] by three defining characteristics of health care that distinguish it from other goods: the unpredictability of need, information asymmetry between patients and providers, and its fundamental importance to people's ability to achieve their life goals. Unpredictability and asymmetry, as the authors recognise, also characterise many other transactions. So we are left with "fundamental importance"—health care as the key to functioning in society—as the key criterion.

This, of course, is unexceptionable: who could disagree? Indeed this criterion is first cousin to the Dunning committee's criterion of "necessity". But how are we to define fundamental importance? The Dunning committee excluded in vitro fertilisation; New and Le Grand consider the inability to have a child to be of fundamental importance. The criterion thus turns out to be vacuous to the extent that it provides no guidance on how conflicting interpretations can be resolved. This leads to a general conclusion: principles that incorporate a semiautomatic formula for implementing them (such as maximising health benefits) tend to be highly contentious, whereas uncontentious principles owe their acceptability to the fact that there is ambiguity about their implementation.

On one point only there appears to be widespread agreement. This is that "ineffective" health care should be excluded from any healthcare package or menu. Again who could disagree? This turns out to be a rather blunt criterion. Most interventions are effective for someone, just as most services may be of fundamental importance to someone. Inevitably attempts at defining a package of health care stub their toes against the rock of patient heterogeneity: a point explored further in the next section.

Problems of practice

Given that it is so difficult to devise coherent criteria or principles, it is not surprising that most attempts to define the healthcare menu have been tentative and somewhat incoherent. The issue has, in effect, been approached backwards: by listing exclusions rather than by defining what is to be included. Oregon remains unique in explicitly setting out what will be provided, as well as what will be excluded—not surprisingly perhaps because the whole venture started as an exercise in extending coverage for the uninsured. Otherwise, however, the problem has been defined, in practice, as an exercise in limiting what is to be available. About a quarter of the 100 health authorities in England explicitly set out, in their purchasing plans for 1996-7, procedures that will not be included in their contracts.[4]

The lists of exclusions are dominated by various forms of cosmetic surgery. These range from tattoo removal to buttock lift, from breast augmentation to procedures for pinning back ears. The reversal of sterilisation and of vasectomy also feature frequently. Also included is in vitro fertilisation. Interestingly, the roll call of exclusions is not some peculiar English eccentricity. Very similar lists have been produced in

Ontario and in Spain when attempts have been made to define entitlements to health care.

Nibbling at the edges

The above catalogue of exclusions is not complete. Health authorities have also begun to exclude some procedures, such as dilatation and curettage for women under 40, where the evidence suggests that they are not clinically effective. But, overall, the exclusions affect only the small change of NHS activity. The implicit criterion appears to be that it is no part of the NHS's responsibilities to deal with conditions that are self inflicted or that can be seen as not being "medical"—that is, as not impairing the ability to function. In effect, it is not the NHS's job to help people to look good.

As a criterion for defining the healthcare menu, this does not take one very far. But the experience of applying even this principle helps to explain why attempts to restrict the menu have been limited to nibbling at the edges—and why, indeed, the whole enterprise is flawed in conception. The pattern is clear. No sooner does a health authority announce that it is proposing not to buy a particular procedure than there is an outcry. In part, this is the reflex reaction of a medical profession that claims that only its members are qualified to pronounce on what patients need. But, more importantly, it reflects the fact of patient heterogeneity. For some patients, if only a very few, even a buttock lift may be crucial for their ability to function socially. Blanket exclusions ignore the fact of patient heterogeneity. Health authorities have therefore tended to retreat from such blanket exclusions to a more flexible position: such procedures are normally not bought unless a clinical need can be demonstrated.

If it is difficult to sustain a policy of blanket exclusions even in the case of marginal procedures, it is not surprising that there has been little or no attempt to extend it to services that make larger demands on the NHS budget and that are more central to people's conception of health care. Much the same conclusion follows if we look at the list of medicines that general practitioners are not permitted to prescribe: these range from various cold relief remedies to toothpaste.[3] Again, the exclusions are conspicuous for their marginality. Any attempt to go further in this direction is therefore likely to mean that there would have to be a disproportionate investment of energy—in terms of persuading professional and public opinion—with a trivial yield in terms of the effects on the NHS's budgetary commitments. And it might well divert attention from the real challenge of managing scarcity in the NHS: which is not whether to provide specific services but how much to provide and how to decide who should be treated and how.

The dimensions of rationing

Explicit rationing through the exclusion of specific procedures or services from the healthcare menu has the great appeal of giving visibility to collective decisions about how the resources devoted to the NHS should be used. But, as argued above, in practice the inevitable price of visibility is triviality. Moreover, any such strategy fails to address the various dimensions of rationing. If rationing is defined as giving patients less demonstrably effective health care than might be desirable in the absence of resource constraints (and from which they would benefit), then it is a pervasive characteristic of the NHS and of other healthcare systems. There is rationing by dilution: offering less intensive care or spending less time with a patient than might be ideal. There is rationing by termination: discharging patients from hospital earlier than desirable. There is rationing by delay: waiting lists are the obvious example.

The following two quotations illustrate the point. The first is from an American commentator on the Oregon experiment:[5]

It takes no great talent to realise that appendectomy is worth funding, at least for a clear cut diagnosis of appendicitis. The real issue is not whether to perform the appendectomy; it is whether to fund countless marginal interventions that are potentially part of the procedure—marginal blood tests and repeat tests; precautionary preventive antibiotic therapy before surgery; the number of nurses in the operating room; and the backup support on call or in the hospital. Even more decisions about marginal elements will arise during the recovery phase; exactly how many days of hospital stay are permitted, how often the physician should make rounds, how many follow up tests there should be, and so on. Many of these are predicted to offer more benefits than harm, but with margins so small that one could argue that resources should be used elsewhere.

The second comes from the Swedish commission on priorities:[1]

If resources are limited then in certain circumstances it may be reasonable to opt for the second best treatment. In hip surgery, for example, a steel prosthesis is less expensive than a titanium one but less durable. It must be considered acceptable for a physician, as is often the case, to choose a steel prosthesis for a patient aged over 80 while giving a titanium one to a patient who is 70 years old and might perhaps need renewed surgery after a few years. In dealing with pronounced coronary strictures involving a risk of stroke, one can choose between surgery and medication. Surgery is a good deal more expensive, involves a short term risk but is in the long term a more effective method of averting stroke. If resources are limited, it may be justifiable to refrain from expanding surgical activities and to stick to medication—which is simple, inexpensive but less effective—instead.

Countless day to day decisions

This, then, is the reality of rationing: countless, day to day decisions by clinicians and others taken in the light of the resources available and the particular circumstances of the patient concerned. Rationing, in effect, is a continuous attempt to reconcile competing claims on limited resources, a balancing act between optimising and satisfying treatment. It is about the exercise of judgment, not about the drawing up of lists of what should or should not be included in the NHS's menu.

Nor is the phenomenon of rationing limited to the acute sector of care. At present there is much debate about the extent to which the NHS should provide long term care and how the demarcation line between social and medical care should be defined. One central fact tends to be overlooked: the NHS has always rationed—to the point of scandal—the care provided in the long term sector. An analysis of the reports of the Health Advisory Service on NHS provision for elderly mentally ill individuals showed that, of the hospitals inspected, 77% had poor sanitary conditions, 66% dilapidated buildings, and 60% overcrowded wards.[6] This is rationing of a very different kind from that discussed previously: the poor quality care flows directly from decisions about the allocation of resources to different parts of the NHS and does not involve clinical decisions. But it is rationing. Dilution could hardly go further.

There are many problems about the kind of implicit rationing that characterises the NHS. It may involve the use of arbitrary and unacceptable criteria, such as the age of the patient. It may mean that the allocation of resources reflects as much the idiosyncrasies of individual clinicians as the characteristics of patients. Clinician heterogeneity is as much of a problem as patient heterogeneity. From this, of course, flows the equity case for defining the care that the NHS should provide. However, it is far from self evident that defining such a package or menu would resolve the equity issue.

Designing a straitjacket

A strict construction of the equity principle would require not only that all health authorities should provide the same range of services but that individual patients should have the same opportunity of getting treatment for any given need. In other words, the argument would move from

91

specifying the range of services to be provided to specifying also the quantity of services to be provided. And indeed there have been some moves in this direction. In the 1980s, the Department of Health started to set health authorities targets for carrying out certain procedures such as coronary artery bypass grafts and hip replacements. For example, the 1990 target was a rate of 300 coronary artery bypass grafts and 1950 hip replacements per million population.[7] Implicit in this strategy was the objective that health authorities should, in effect, deliver a particular quantity of specified packages of health care to their populations. This strategy appears to have been largely abandoned as the Department's focus has switched to outcomes, but it shows that, in principle at least, it would be possible to define both the menu and the number of meals to be served.

Indeed the equity case for designing a basic package of care would seem to require taking this further step. For without it "inconsistency and arbitrariness in the rationing of health care", as New and Le Grand put it, would surely persist. In vitro fertilisation provides an illustration. Many health authorities have decided against excluding this from their provision but have, instead, adopted a strategy of limiting the number of procedures to be made available. They therefore ration by the selection of patients, with different health authorities using different criteria (the age of the prospective mother, the stability of the partnership, etc) for selecting candidates. The service actually provided could therefore be extremely sparse and largely symbolic in many areas. And while in vitro fertilisation may be a special case, differences in the way in which health authorities interpret their responsibilities are in no way exceptional. Throughout the whole range of NHS provision variation in the level of services provided is the norm.

Pursuing the logic

Advocates of specifying the range of service to be provided by the NHS tend, however, to flinch from the logic of their own arguments. Thus New and Le Grand (to quote, again, the most sophisticated exponents of this approach) conclude that although every health authority would have to provide at least some level of service for the specified range "the actual level of provision, highly contingent on local circumstances, would be left to local discretion". So "inconsistency and arbitrariness" come in by the back door of local discretion.

There is, of course, a case for local discretion. The scope for substitution in health care is great: a deficit in one kind of service may be compensated for by provision elsewhere. Health care is in a continuous process of technological and organisational evolution and to specify particular levels of service would put the NHS in a straitjacket, inhibiting adaptation and innovation. The concept of "need" is, itself, highly elusive, and flexibility in its interpretation is essential. However much we may chafe at the way in which local discretion is often exercised, it still seems preferable to imposing a national template on the design and delivery of health care.

But if this line of argument is accepted, there is little left of the case for devising an NHS menu. If its proponents refuse to accept the full logic of their own case—if they rightly recoil from the notion of imposing a national template on the NHS—there would seem little point in travelling half way down the road with them. Rather than worrying about drawing up an NHS menu, we should concentrate on what is going on in the kitchen: we should accept the inevitability and indeed desirability of leaving rationing decisions to clinicians and concentrate on ways of making the profession collectively more accountable for the way in which they carry out this onerous task.

1 Klein R, Day P, Redmayne S. *Managing scarcity: priority setting and rationing in the NHS.* Buckingham: Open University Press, 1996.
2 Redmayne S, Klein R. Rationing in practice: the case of in vitro fertilisation. *BMJ* 1993: 306:1521-4.
3 New B, Le Grand J. *Rationing in the NHS: principles and pragmatism.* London: King's Fund, 1996.
4 Redmayne S. *Small steps, big goals: purchasing policies in the NHS.* Birmingham: NAHAT, 1996.
5 Veatch RM. The Oregon experiment: needless and real worries. In: Strosberg MA, Wiener JM, Baker R, Fein IA, eds. *Rationing America's medical care: The Oregon plan and beyond.* Washington, DC: Brookings Institution, 1992.
6 Day P, Klein R, Tipping G. *Inspecting for quality: services for the elderly.* Bath: Centre for the Study of Social Policy, 1988.
7 Department of Health and Office of Population Censuses and Surveys. *Departmental Report.* London: HMSO, 1992 (Cm 1913).

A rejoinder to Rudolf Klein

BILL NEW

Rudolf Klein offers a very fair critique of the proposals set out in "Devising a health care package: the case for", and in most respects, although I stand by my arguments, the judgment on the relative merits of the two positions must now rest with the reader. However, on one particular matter, I believe that he does do something of an injustice to the arguments presented.

Part of the case for devising a package rests on a novel method for establishing what should be included in it. Instead of relying on the traditional methods of establishing cost effectiveness or making ill defined

93

judgments about what constitutes "health", I (along with Julian Le Grand in the original book[1]) proposed that one should instead refer to the characteristics that make health care unsuitable for market exchange in the first place. If those characteristics are present then the service should be part of the NHS package. Quoting Klein:

> Public provision or financing is justified, New and Le Grand argue, by three defining characteristics of health care that distinguish it from other goods: the unpredictability of need, information asymmetry between patients and providers and its fundamental importance to people's ability to achieve their life goals. Unpredictability and asymmetry, as the authors recognise, also characterise many other transactions. So we are left with "fundamental importance"—health care as the key to functioning in society—as the key criterion.
>
> This, of course, is unexceptionable: who could disagree? . . .

It is the concluding sentence of this passage that, I believe, somewhat misrepresents our position. Perhaps no one would disagree that fundamental importance is an important criterion, but it is not the key criterion, let alone the only one. It is the combination of all three criteria that sets health care apart. There are, in fact, many other goods and services that are of fundamental importance—food and clothing, for example—but they are not financed on a universal basis by the state. Instead, income transfers are effected such that people can afford these fundamental goods, and the market then operates in a perfectly satisfactory way to provide them. In short, there is no market failure caused by information imbalance and uncertainty.

Of course, there is a need for further judgment on whether the criteria are satisfied. But at the very least they remind us that "fundamental importance" alone is not sufficient reason for the state to finance a service on a universal basis. And at best they may provide a helpful guide in making the tricky decisions about the boundary of NHS responsibility. When viewed in this way they look significantly less bland than at first sight.

1 New B, Le Grand J. *Rationing in the NHS: principles and pragmatism.* London: King's Fund, 1996.

7 Maximising the health of the whole community

The principal objective of the NHS ought to be to maximise the aggregate improvement in the health status of the whole community

The case for

TONY CULYER

Caveats

It seems a pity to compromise what seems uncompromising, but let us begin with some health warnings.

First, "principal" does not mean "only", and some of the other things the NHS does (and ought to do) turn out to be necessary anyway if it is to achieve this prime objective. Moreover, efficiency (which is what maximising is about) needs always to be tempered by consideration of equity in both process and outcome.

Second, let's remind ourselves that most moral objectives (of which this is one) do not lose their force by virtue of being impossible to attain—one of the reasons for having moral rules about anything is that they provide bases for judging how well is doing with respect to what one ought to be doing.

Third, let's remember that there are good reasons for our having taken health care out of the "ordinary" market place. These include: a solidarity type case that ensures no one is excluded from benefit on grounds of lack of portable, transparent, and comprehensive entitlement; protection from professional dominance in the determination of both general healthcare priorities and specific patient–doctor relations (in any system of health care it is primarily the doctor who determines the demand for care, not the patient); equity in funding arrangements, processes, and outcome (mainly health); and the provision of care that is more likely to confer benefit than harm.

Fourth, maximising such an objective involves not only a commitment to the ethicality of that which is being maximised, but also embodies within it a host of other ethical issues; these often take the form of trade offs,

95

whose exposure, discussion, and resolution by people with legitimate rights to be involved is important.

Fifth, maximising anything implies the need for particular sorts of knowledge: for information about health status, changes in it, its decomposition into relevant population subgroups, and believable attribution of such changes to causes (whether they lie in the delivery of health care or through other means).

Finally, the desirability of measurement in general ought to be distinguished from the suitability and acceptability of any specific measure. One desideratum of any measure of health or health gain is that it should enable interpersonal comparisons of health gain (or loss) to be made; this is one of the striking departures from the more general utilitarian objectives customarily set by economists in evaluating the advantages and disadvantages of various institutions and policy options. A common objection to health measurement is not so much an objection to outcome measurement itself as to either a particular measure of it (for example, that it misses something important out) or to a particular way of using a measure (for example, not weighting prospective health gain, or prospective health gainers, differentially according to morally relevant factors). One of the attractions of explicit measures of prospective outcome is that they clearly expose sins of commission and omission. Thus, they enable the explicit discussion and implementation of equity based desiderata, rather than leaving them to the uninformed whim of individuals and committees with influence.

NHS ought to be about maximising health

There can be no doubt that a principal objective of the NHS is to maximise health. We have ministerial authority for that. The more interesting, non-factual assertion is that it ought to do this. The ethical underpinnings for my view are that it ought lie in the importance of good health for people to lead flourishing lives, which I take as an ultimate good. We can all think of individuals with terrible handicaps of ill health who seem to flourish but these are not persuasive counter examples. Such people excite our admiration and are seen as exceptional.

In general, I take it that flourishing is an ultimate good and that good health is in general a necessary condition for achieving this ultimate good. In short, health is needed in the twin senses that it is both necessary (just as my possessing a Rolls-Royce is a necessary sign of my personal success in life) and serves an ethically commendable end. This gives an otherwise merely technical relationship between means and ends its ethically persuasive quality and raises the need for health to high ethical significance (in a way that is not true for my need for a "roller").

96

To take the argument further, health care (including medical care) may be a necessary (though not sufficient) condition for realising better health. If so, it too is needed (that is, is necessary if improved health is to be attained) and it too derives its ethically compelling character from the ethicality of the flourishing that is the ultimate good. So, not only may it be reasonably assumed that individuals want health care; they also need it in an ethically persuasive sense of the word.

If all that is accepted, maximising the health of populations becomes an ethical objective, as does being efficient so that the resources used in health care are used to maximise health outcomes. This is not the same as maximising the use of beneficial health care—or effectiveness. It differs from it principally in that delivering only that care which is most effective takes no account of the opportunity cost of such care (a highly effective but very costly treatment may rightly be given lower priority than a less effective but much cheaper one) when both cannot be delivered to all who might benefit. Distributive justice also acquires a high priority: in my view (which is not that equity is sufficiently served by maximising some equity weighted outcome measure) this is best tackled in terms of seeking to identify and move towards a more equal distribution of health across the population while at the same time ensuring that each procedure offered to patients is that believed (on the best evidence available) to be the most cost effective. This will not usually imply an equal distribution of resources, nor will it imply a curmudgeonly equality in which everyone gets nothing (equally). It actually implies, given current knowledge of the way medical technology is deployed, both a rise in the average health of people and a more equal distribution of health. There are twin problems for social decision makers here. One (for healthcare commissioners and providers) is the selective use of their resources to achieve objectives efficiently. Others (for higher level decision makers) involve trading off other ultimately good things which we might legitimately seek in pursuit of flourishing lives but which compete with health care in the battle for resources. There is no room for absolutism here, for there is more than one means to the great ethical end of flourishing. Nor can every desirable thing be done for everyone. Conflict, and the need to choose, is inevitable.

Efficiency and equity aren't always in opposition

Conflicts can, however, be overdone. One that is commonly overdone is the alleged clash between efficiency and equity. If we define efficiency in a health service as being the maximisation of probable health outcomes, and there is also an acceptable quantification of these outcomes across the variety of activity we call "health services", then there exists, as a matter of logic, such a maximum for every possible distribution of resources to

97

individuals. All these possible distributions are efficient. But all are most certainly not fair or equitable. Choosing between these possible distributions, all of which are efficient, cannot involve any conflict between efficiency and equity—unless you make the additional ethical judgment that the marginal unit of outcome is always of equal value to whomsoever it accrues. I see no compelling moral argument for such a judgment.

Talking theoretically, although difficult, can sound glib. In practice one is in a sea of uncertainty, even in a world as conceptually simple as that just described. There is a deficit of usable relevant information on health itself, its distribution across population groups, on health gains (actual or projected), on the links between the activities of the NHS and their final impact on people's health, on the reasons for the huge variations that can be measured between practitioners and the variations in outcomes that individual practitioners achieve. As a practical example, the enormous clinically inexplicable variations in general practitioners' referrals within and across health authority areas are a source of both deep inequity and substantial inefficiency which only health authorities can address.

For many in the research and development commissioning communities, these lacunae provide the (ethical) momentum for changes that have recently been set in train in the research and development programme, for the intelligent use of evidence based medicine, for outcome measurement, and for the partial separation of the activity of healthcare commissioning from healthcare delivery. There is an act of faith involved here, which is that more evidence relating to the components of the links in the flourishing healthcare cascade is a good thing. This involves a belief that more (relevant) information is better than less and a commitment to the principle that the best should not be allowed to become the enemy of the good.

Information not a substitute for judgment

Undoubtedly, the mere provision of information is insufficient—at the very least it will need interpretation in particular contexts by patients and professionals who understand enough of its limitations not to fall into the trap of supposing that information can ever be a substitute for judgment (including clinical judgment). Moreover, there is abundant evidence that the mere provision of even very good information is not itself sufficient to get the professionals to act on it. Further, issues of value pervade the entire decision structure. At one level it is impossible to define "health" without value judgments (whose should they be?); at another, it is usually impossible to determine the appropriate course of medical actions for a particular patient without making patient specific value judgments (whose, again, should these be?). There are values to be selected at all points in between.

98

As I wrote at the beginning, improved health is not the only business of the NHS. In relations with patients a common task in both primary and secondary care is to provide information—and no more: information that a person does not have the disease he or she feared, about whom outside the NHS to contact for help with a problem, about healthy lifestyles, and so on. Plainly, such information serves an ethical end. Moreover, it may also serve the end of health maximisation—health education, for example. The institutional side of the NHS also provides hotel services, which ought to be provided efficiently but which may not raise questions of distributive equity of the same compelling sort as does active medical care itself and might be left to private purchasing power and insurance arrangements without damaging the objectives of the NHS.

Similarly, equity in the distribution of health (or of health gain, or of healthcare resources) does not exhaust what ought to be proper equity concerns in the NHS. Procedures and processes too must be fair. It is not fair: to keep similarly placed people waiting avoidably different times; for professionals to be rude or inconsiderate; to treat professionals within the system as though they were employees in a command economy, or to set them professional targets without also supplying the means by which they might meet them; or to exclude those for whom the NHS exists from decisions about the values that are to be incorporated in the layers of this many tiered cake.

Work on measures is needed

Setting an objective of the sort postulated here is not the usual way that economists have approached issues of efficiency and equity. They have more usually had a particular and rather sophisticated branch of utilitarianism to set the conceptual rules for resource allocation which goes under the name "Paretian welfare economics". This is the view that decisions ought to maximise subjectively perceived welfare, that the only identifiable improvements are those where no one loses such welfare and at least one gains some, and that in situations where some gain and others lose one can only sit on one's hands. Some of us have rejected this framework for health and health care not because we want to reject the respect for individual values which is enshrined within its ethical frame but because it fails to deliver practical guidelines with practical consequences and, where it does, does so with severe limitations. A particular weakness of the traditional Paretian approach is that it affords no leverage on choices that have to be made which involve some people losing while others gain—which is, sadly, the usual situation. The usual evaluative framework is also silent for choices that are based on considerations of equity.

This is not true of the object set here (maximising health) provided that a suitable measure of the thing to be maximised is available. Twenty five years ago no such measure was available. That is no longer true. A battery of claimants exists, each of which has its advantages and disadvantages and some of which may be more appropriate to some types of choice than others. We need appropriate measures for all the outputs of the NHS that are of prime concern and indicators of the varied dimensions that equity takes. We also need a community of users of this information who can interpret and use it towards the NHS's objective and who can feed problems back to the consumer and the professional, managerial, and research communities so that improvements and refinements can be made and lacunae filled. All this entails comprehensive partnerships and dialogue across a spectrum of communities and interest groups. It also requires education, training, and research.

The practical problem at all levels of the NHS is to be able to apply consistent and acceptable principles to answer questions like: Which services shall be available? To whom shall they be available? On what conditions shall they be available? These questions are all rationing questions, and the principles need to be practically useful and defensible by those who use them. If you don't find mine acceptable (at least they meet the requirements of consistency and applicability and are derived from a set of explicit ethical considerations), then what are your alternatives—and how would you expect ministers, the NHS Executive, NHS managers, and NHS professionals to implement them?

The case against (what the principal objective of the NHS should really be)

JOHN HARRIS

Patients rationally want three things from health care. They want the treatment that will give them maximum life expectancy coupled with the best quality of that life, and above all they want the best possible opportunity of getting the combination of quantity and quality of life available to them given their personal health status. I believe that each citizen has an equal claim on the protection of the community as expressed by its public health care system, and this means that each is entitled to an equal chance of

100

having his or her, necessarily individual, health needs respected by any publicly funded healthcare system.

Means and ends

It is common ground I suppose that we have to think about the ethics both of means and of ends. Even if it were to be accepted that the healthcare system ought principally to aim at maximising aggregate health gain, it does not follow that the most effective ways of achieving this are legitimate. If all seriously ill people were to be allowed to die this might dramatically improve the aggregate health of the community at large. I hope such a policy would not seem ethically defensible. Yet this is precisely what measures which use quality adjusted life years, or similar mechanisms, do: they systematically accord preference to those who have better health prospects, and, by selecting against those with worse prospects, tend to improve the aggregate health status of the whole community at the expense of the life chances of those with poorer prognosis.

We should notice that to make aggregate improvements a principal objective, even if not the only objective, is to imply the subordination of the health needs of individuals to something very abstract, and in some circumstances something very trivial indeed—namely, the improved health status of the whole community. For this could imply sacrificing the life of one person who was very ill and expensive to treat, if doing so would make even a tiny improvement to the aggregate health status, an improvement which no individual would even notice.

Distributive justice

Distributive justice must be built into any articulation of principal objectives for the NHS, but it cannot be enough to define the relevant principle of distributive justice in terms of a more equal distribution of health across populations, because such an objective could be achieved as much by levelling down as by levelling up. One method of allocating a scarce resource which apparently satisfies the requirements of justice is, of course, not to allocate that resource to anyone. All are then treated equally.

The fallacy of such a supposition is easily illustrated. The principles of justice, and indeed the principles of equality, are moral principles, principles that are designed to be more than impartial, that are designed among other things to respect and to do justice to people. In some sense this must involve some benevolent attitude to people which is often abbreviated as "respect for persons". Such an attitude to others is as different as it is

101

possible to be to that of simply showing an equality of lack of respect or an equal indifference to their fate.

So, neither the failure to allocate resources that would save lives or protect individuals nor the simple attempt to move towards a more equal distribution of health could be part of a claim to satisfy the requirements of equality or justice conceived of as moral principles (and how else are we to think of them?). This is because equality or distributive justice has at its heart the claim that people's lives and fundamental interests are of value, that they matter. Anyone who denied resources which would protect life and other fundamental interests is not valuing the lives of those to whom she denies these protections. Although she might be treating people equally in the sense of treating them all the same, she is not treating them as equals, as people who matter and hence matter equally.

Now this brings us close to the positive part of my account, because I believe it to be an integral part of any principle of distributive justice that people's moral claims to resources are not diminished by who they are; how old they are; how rich or poor, powerful or weak, they are; or by the quality of their lives. A principle of justice worth its salt covers young and old, healthy and sick, weak and strong, regardless of race, creed, colour, sex, quality of life, and life expectancy. Before further articulating the basis of this principle and what it means for the objectives of the NHS we must take a brief look at the concept of efficiency.

Efficiency

Efficiency in the delivery of health care is often defined in terms of maximising beneficial health care or of maximising health outcomes. These styles of definition of efficiency simply beg the question at issue. This question is: what is the good to be delivered by health care? They beg the question because they imply that the greater the health gain per treatment the greater the efficiency of that treatment. This implication is true in one context or application but false in another and it is the conflation of applications, either negligently or deliberately, which gives such plausibility as it has to the proposition that the NHS ought principally to maximise aggregate improvements in health status.

It is true that in order sensibly to maximise health outcomes you need an acceptable measure of success or failure. However, prioritising those outcomes you can best measure and calling it "maximisation of health outcomes" is letting the tail wag the dog. Any measure of what health care tries to maximise which counts life years after treatment faces a problem. The problem turns on the difference between selecting between different treatments for the same patient and selecting between different patients for the same treatment.

102

This distinction is of the first importance. If you are choosing between rival therapies for the same condition you would be wise to choose the therapy which maximises health outcomes. However, it is a fallacy to suppose that the measure of what is the best or most efficient treatment for a particular patient or condition can also be the measure of the most efficient or best way of distributing resources for care among patients when this amounts to prioritising patients for treatment rather than treatments for patients. The question of which is the most efficient treatment for this patient or condition is not the same as the question: which patients or groups of patients is it efficient or beneficial to treat? This is because there is an equivocation over the meaning of "beneficial" in the two contexts and a problem about incompatible ways of quantifying the size of benefit.

Incompatible approaches

If the millionaire and the pauper both lose all they have in the stock market crash, in one way of thinking about the loss, each has suffered the same degree of loss, each has lost everything. In another, each has suffered a different quantity of loss measured by the total sum lost. There is no straightforward way of reconciling these different approaches. If we are searching for an equitable approach to loss it is not obvious that we should devote resources allocated to loss minimisation to ensuring that the millionaire is protected rather than the pauper. The same is true of health gain. Even if it is agreed that resources devoted to health care are resources devoted to minimising the loss of health or maximising the health gain, it could not be demonstrated that the person who stands to lose more life years if they die prematurely stands to suffer a greater loss than the person who has less life expectancy. Nor can it be shown that the measure of health gain must equate to the number of life years, quality adjusted or not, which flow from treatment.

If you and I are competitors for treatment and I will have a better health outcome from treatment than you, but both of us will make a health gain that is significant and important to us, automatically preferring to satisfy my needs rather than yours seems unfair. Why should my life be judged more worth saving because I am more healthy rather than more intelligent, say, or more useful? Arguments can (and have) been made on both sides, but to define need, for example, in terms of capacity to benefit and then argue that the greater the number of life years deliverable by health care, the greater the need for treatment (or the greater the patient's interest in receiving treatment) is just to beg the crucial question of how to characterise need or benefit.

Equally, to define efficiency in terms of "the maximisation of health outcomes" and then argue that efficiency demands that the NHS aims at maximising aggregate health gain across the whole community is just to beg the question as to how we should think of the gain or benefit to be delivered by the NHS. Efficiency is like motherhood and apple pie; no one can admit to being against it. Arguably health outcomes are maximised and a healthcare system operates efficiently when more people who can derive significant benefit from it are given their chance of access to health care.

I suggested at the start that patients want the treatment that will give them maximum life expectancy coupled with the best quality of that life and the best possible opportunity of getting the combination of quantity and quality of life available to them. Maximising aggregate improvements in health status of the whole community will not necessarily be a rational strategy for achieving these three objectives. Whether it is or not will depend on one's existing or probable health status. This in turn will depend on many things, including one's genetic constitution. If one principal aim of the NHS ought to be to give the people it serves what they want for themselves then this is unlikely to be the maximisation of aggregate improvements in health status. People tend to want the best for themselves and those they care most about, and a policy aimed at maximising aggregate improvements in health status will tend to favour those with the best prospects of large improvements, those with a "healthy" genome for example. People would only be likely to choose such a policy if they could be sure that they themselves would likely benefit.

NHS is there to protect life and liberty

Imagine an industrialised state that has big conurbations where millions of citizens are concentrated, many smaller towns, and thousands of tiny villages. It has vast sparsely populated tracts of agricultural land and vaster mountainous areas and wilderness where few people live. How should it distribute its access to health care? Probably it will place the major hospitals and medical schools in the centres of population, but smaller hospitals and medical centres will serve the smaller towns and isolated villages. For the remotest areas there will probably be an air rescue service or even a flying doctor or flying hospital service.

For geographical reasons if for no other, those in the most remote regions will be generally more expensive to treat. To fly the remote farmer and backwoodsman to the major centres of excellence for specialised treatment will be naturally more costly and hence less cost effective than to bus suburban commuters downtown. We will assume, what is probably true, that the funds devoted to servicing the health needs of citizens who are geographically remote from major centres would have treated more people had they been allocated to urban populations. Why do societies divert

104

resources available for health care away from the more numerous city dwellers in a way which must adversely affect their ability to maximise aggregate improvements in health status or indeed to maximise numbers treated?

I believe the ends subserved by public healthcare systems are broadly the same as those which justify the high priority given to national defence. All governments and would be governments boast the strongest commitment to national defence. The question that is seldom asked is what is national defence for, what justifies its prominent place in national priorities? The simplistic answer is, of course, that without national defence there might be no nation and hence no national priorities. But pressed further it is reasonable to ask for the underlying values and interests it subserves.

Equal protection

Arguably protecting citizens against threats to their lives, liberties, and fundamental interest is the first priority for any state. When in 1651 Thomas Hobbes wrote "The obligation of subjects to the sovereign, is understood to last as long, and no longer, than the power lasteth, by which he is able to protect them" he was providing an answer to this question. On this view, any citizen's obligation to the state and to obey its laws is conditional on the state for its part protecting that citizen against threats to his or her life and liberty. If we reflect on what citizens today want and need in the way of protection I believe we will find that in most contemporary societies the most important threats to life and liberty come not in the form of soldiers with snow on their boots but from illness, accident, and poverty. This is why it is arguable that the obligation to provide health care, and in particular life saving health care, to each and every citizen, regardless of its effect on the aggregate health status of the community, takes precedence over the obligation to provide defence forces against external (and often mythical) enemies.

There is a good principle which states that real and present dangers should be met before future and speculative ones. If this is right the healthcare system should have first claim on the national defence budget. I should make clear that no part of my argument assumes a given budget for health care; rather I argue that the budget could and should be larger, that the health budget has first call on the defence budget, but that whatever the budget is, there are ways of distributing the budget which are to be avoided because they are unjust.

Another feature of the state's obligation to defend its citizens which is often overlooked is its egalitarian nature. Just as each citizen owes his or her obligation to obey the law regardless of such features as race, religion, sex or age, quality of life, or prognosis, so the state must discharge its obligation of protection with the same impartiality. If we expect people to obey the law even though their life expectancy is short and the quality of their life poor, we must not deny them the equal protection that is an essential part of the social contract. I have suggested that the protection of the healthcare system is one of the principal elements of the state's side of this contract and that discrimination against those with poor quality of life or shorter life expectancy in the allocation of such resources is a betrayal, not only of those citizens, but of the social contract. Where all cannot be treated and priorities must be set the basis of prioritisation should not be the effect on the aggregate health of the whole community, for this will tend to discriminate against those arguably most in need of health care.

The principal objective of the NHS should be to protect the life and health of each citizen impartially and to offer beneficial health care on the basis of individual need, so that each has an equal chance of flourishing to the extent that their personal health status permits.

A rejoinder to John Harris

TONY CULYER

I agree with Harris's ending: the NHS should give each "an equal chance of flourishing", but would add "subject to the availability of NHS resources and the potential each has to flourish". He would reject this because the NHS's budget should be larger (again I agree)—sufficiently large to exhaust all citizen's "wants" (I disagree). He does not address the issues raised by people having different capabilities of flourishing. He begins by guessing (no evidence is offered) what patients "rationally" want. I don't know what work the qualifier "rational" is doing. He talks about "needs" (without differentiating them from mere "wants"; people may want what they do not need and need what they do not want) and says that all are entitled to have needs "respected" (ought not wants to be respected too, and does "respect" entail "must be met"?), thus avoiding the question of what is to be done when resources are insufficient to meet all wants (or, come to that, needs). The implication is that resources should be available to meet the smallest want/need. In short, he bypasses the central issue by assuming away the problem generating the necessity of "rationing". Moreover, he believes that health care wants trump (all?) others, certainly defence wants (as though these too had no contribution to make to "flourishing"). At

106

the one point where scarcity gets a mention—end of the penultimate paragraph—we are told only what the rationing criterion ought not to be. I do not see much in all this to help us design or manage a better NHS. There are confusions. One muddles need for health and need for health care. To "flourish" one arguably needs health but if health care can do nothing for one's health, it cannot be needed (that is, it cannot be necessary for "flourishing").

Efficiency is not the same as "the greatest gain per treatment" either for individuals or across them. Efficiency exists when you cannot improve the health of one within NHS resources without reducing that of another. It does not imply people in remote areas getting fewer NHS resources (other things being equal). You can posit any number of geographical carve ups of NHS funding you like and for each there will be an efficient result—that is, for each distribution there will be a maximum population health gain. Each is equally efficient. The efficiency principle gives no indication of which carve up is best. For that you need a principle of geographical or interpersonal equity. There is no conflict between efficiency and equity! Efficiency alone is insufficient for decisions. Equity principles enable choice between efficient allocations but neither are they sufficient. We need both types of principle.

The assertion that outcome measures based on future life-years entail allowing all seriously ill people to die is logically wrong (as well as immoral). Measurement itself entails few consequences, although the use of bad measures or the misuse of good ones might. Nor does someone being very ill signal a need for health care. Three things matter: prospective health gain from health care (which may be very good even if one is very old or sick now, or poor even if one is quite young or well now); an acceptable measure of it; and the opportunity cost of achieving it—the loss of prospective health for others by using resources for one patient rather than others.

I would "sacrifice" the life of one person for whom health care could do nothing to save the lives of others for whom care can do much, or others whose (say) elderly lives are not at risk but are blighted by arthritic hips but for whom extremely cost effective technologies exist. This is not really a sacrifice at all: offering health care to that patient will not help her or him anyway. But extreme cases are not very interesting, because the opportunity cost of health care for these others is, by definition, zero.

8 Rationing health care by age

Age is an appropriate criterion for choosing which people who could benefit from health care should be offered it

The case for

ALAN WILLIAMS

As we grow older our recuperative powers diminish. Thus we accumulate a distressing collection of chronic incurable conditions. Some of these are no more than a minor nuisance, and we adapt as best we can; and when adaptation is not possible we learn to tolerate them. Some are more serious, involving severe disability and persistent pain, and may eventually become life threatening.

We are also at risk of various acute conditions (like influenza or pneumonia) which are more serious threats to the health of elderly people than to younger people. We also have more difficulty recovering from what younger people would regard as minor injuries (such as falls). When you add to all this the increased likelihood that illness (and other disruptions of our normal lifestyle) will leave us rather confused and in need of more rehabilitative and social support than a young person, it is hardly surprising that NHS expenditure per person rises sharply after about age 65.

The vain pursuit of immortality

People are also living longer, and people aged over 65 now form a much bigger proportion of the population than they used to. From the viewpoint of NHS expenditure this would not matter if the extra years of life were predominantly healthy years but it would if the extra years were ones of disability, pain, and increasing dependence on others.

The evidence on this is ambiguous. Many people remain fit and independent well into their 80s. Others enter their 60s already afflicted with the aftermath of stroke, heart disease, arthritis, or bronchitis. It is not clear whether things are getting worse at each year of age, or whether

108

expectations are rising and people are now more likely to report disabilities once shrugged off as the inevitable consequence of getting old. That many of these conditions are incurable does not mean they are untreatable. Much can be done to reduce their adverse consequences, including many remedial activities which lie outside the NHS (such as home adaptations, domestic support, and special accommodation).

It is important to get away from the notion of "cure" as the criterion of benefit and adopt instead measures of effectiveness that turn on the impact of treatments on people's health related quality of life. Such an approach concentrates on the features that people themselves value, such as mobility, self care, being able to pursue usual activities (whatever they are), and being free of pain and discomfort and anxiety and depression.

Improving the quality of life of elderly people in these ways may not be very costly, but these unglamorous down to earth activities tend to lose out to high tech interventions which gain their emotional hold by claiming that life threatening conditions should always take priority. This vain pursuit of immortality is dangerous for elderly people: taken to its logical conclusion it implies that no one should be allowed to die until everything possible has been done. That means not simply that we shall all die in hospital but that we shall die in intensive care.

Reasonable limits

This attempt to wring the last drop of medical benefit out of the system, no matter what the human and material costs, is not the hallmark of a humane society. In each of our lives there has to come a time when we accept the inevitability of death, and when we also accept that a reasonable limit has to be set on the demands we can properly make on our fellow citizens in order to keep us going a bit longer.

It would be better for that limit to be set, with fairly general consent, before we as individuals get into that potentially harrowing situation. When the time comes we shall probably each want an exception made in our case, because few of us are strong willed enough to act cheerfully in the general public interest when our own welfare is at stake. But if a limit is to be set, on what principles should it be determined? And what is their justification? And what role does age have?

In arguing for this chapter's proposition I have sought to make two contextual points clear: first, that ability to benefit should be measured in rather broader terms than cure or survival and, second, that although chronological age is the best single predictor of increasing health problems, it is only a predictor, not a mechanistic determinant.

But age as an indicator of declining recuperative powers, of future health problems, of increasing need for health care, and of declining capacity to

109

benefit from health care (because of shorter life expectancy) is only half the story. It addresses the issue of whether age is a good indicator of the extent to which people could benefit from health care but not in itself of whether they should be offered it. This more crucial step depends on what the objectives of the NHS are to be.

The NHS's objectives

If we start with the proposition that the objective should be to improve as much as possible the health of the nation as a whole then the people who should get priority are those who will benefit most from the resources available. In some cases the old will benefit most, in others the young. But for treatments that yield benefits that last for the rest of a person's life (or for a long time) the young will generally benefit more, because the rest of a young person's life is usually longer than the rest of an old person's life. And even among old people themselves the life expectancy of a 70 year old is usually greater than that of an 80 year old. Where a treatment offers only modest benefits a person may have to live a long time to make treatment worth while—that is, to make the benefit to that person larger than the sacrifices of rival candidates who failed to get treated. So improving the health of the nation as a whole is likely, in some circumstances, to discriminate indirectly against older people.

Is this morally defensible? Well, if we behaved otherwise we would by implication be asserting that in order to provide small benefits for elderly people, young people should sacrifice large benefits. What makes old people more deserving of health benefits than young people? One argument might be that all their lives they have been paying their taxes to finance the healthcare system (among other things), and just when they need health care most the government lets them down. But the government—that is, their fellow citizens—did not promise to do everything possible no matter what the costs.

The NHS is part of a social insurance system, not a savings club for each individual's health care expenditures. It is the lucky ones who do not get their money's worth out of the system, and the unlucky ones who need heavy NHS expenditures all their lives. The NHS is there to meet certain contingencies but not others. And many of the treatments that the NHS now offers to old people in certain contingencies were not even invented when they started contributing 40 or 50 years ago. So to argue, from a historical viewpoint, about an entitlement to get your money's worth seems inappropriate to any insurance scheme, and in particular to a social insurance scheme such as the NHS.

A different line of argument might be that as the number of years left becomes smaller and smaller, each is more precious. The implication of

110

this argument is that elderly people value their small improvements more highly than young people do their much larger improvements. This raises a fundamental problem about whose values should count in a social insurance setting. Suppose that it were true that older people would spend relatively more on health care to get health improvements rather than other things, whereas younger people would spend relatively more on (say) education for their children and rather less on health benefits for themselves. Rational self interest drives individual citizens operating in private markets precisely in that direction.

But did we not take the NHS out of that context precisely because as citizens (rather than as consumers of health care) we were pursuing a rather different ideal—namely, that health care should be provided according to people's needs, not according to what they were each willing and able to pay. A person's needs (constituting claims on social resources) have to be arbitrated by a third party, whose unenviable task it is to weigh different needs (and different people's needs) one against another. This is precisely what priority setting in health care is all about. So the values of the citizenry as a whole must override the values of a particular interest group within it.

A fair innings

So I can find no compelling argument to justify the view that the young should sacrifice large benefits so that the old can enjoy small ones. But I can find an argument which goes in the opposite direction. It is that one of the objectives of the healthcare system should be to reduce inequalities in people's lifetime experience of health. The popular folklore is rich in phrases indicating that we all have some vague notion of a "fair innings" in health terms. Put at its crudest, it reflects the biblical idea that the years of our life are three score and ten. Anyone who achieves or exceeds this is reckoned to have had a fair innings, whereas anyone who dies at an earlier age "was cut off in their prime" or "died tragically young". As has been observed, although it is always a misfortune to die if you wish to go on living, it is both a misfortune and a tragedy to die young. Why?

From my perspective (approaching the age of 70) I see clearly why it is a tragedy, because someone who dies young has been denied the opportunities that we older people have already had. If reducing inequalities in lifetime health is a worthy social objective, it will lead us to be willing to do more to enable young people to survive than we are willing to do to enable old people to survive.

But I do not think that the notion of a "fair innings" should be restricted to matters of survival and life expectancy. Quality of life considerations concerning health may be just as important. Someone who has suffered a

111

lifetime of pain and disability cannot be said to have had a fair innings even if she did live to be 80, and I would therefore extend the concept to embrace something more than just years of life. My preferred concept would be the number of quality adjusted life years a person had enjoyed. On the whole people's earlier years are healthy years, and their later years less healthy years, so this does not affect the general tenor of my argument. What it implies is that we need to consider, alongside age itself, the quality of a person's lifetime experience of health. The worse it has been, the more consideration they deserve, age for age.

Age matters

So my overall conclusion is that age matters in two respects. First, it affects people's capacity to benefit, and therefore places them at a general disadvantage if the objective is to maximise the benefits of health care. Second, the older you are the more likely you will have achieved what your fellow citizens would judge to have been a fair innings, and this will place old people at a disadvantage if the objective is to minimise the differences in lifetime experience of health. I would be the first to admit that I personally have had a fair innings and that it would not be equitable to deny a younger person large benefits in order to provide small ones for me. Indeed, I would go further: it would be equitable to provide small benefits for a young person even if by so doing I were denied large benefits, provided that the young person in question had a low probability of ever achieving a fair innings. Note that this argument does not mean that benefits to young people take absolute priority over benefits to old people. It simply means that we give rather more weight to them than to us.

Surveys of public opinion commonly find that most people, if pushed into a tight situation, would give priority to the young over the old when distributing a given amount of healthcare benefit. There is also little doubt that healthcare professionals share this general attitude. It does not, of course, stop them from being kind, considerate, and caring when old people need health care, but it manifests itself at the level of clinical policy making, when different needs have to be prioritised. For the professionals what may be in their minds may be mostly old people's impaired capacity to benefit from health care. But I strongly suspect that some variant of the fair innings argument also underlies such views, and this is especially likely to be the case among the general public. When the views of older respondents in such surveys have been reported separately, they too give priority to the young over themselves.

So I am encouraged to hope that, in the interests of fairness between the generations, the members of my generation will exercise restraint in the demands we make on the healthcare system. We should not object to age being one of the criteria (though not the sole criterion) used in the prioritisation of health care, even though it will disadvantage us. The alternative is too outrageous to contemplate—namely, that we expect the young to make large sacrifices so that we can enjoy small benefits. That would not be fair.

A rejoinder to Alan Williams

JOHN GRIMLEY EVANS

Those who are daily immersed in the realities of the NHS have a different view of its working from those who never have to smell blood or fear. Of course, there have been horror stories from the USA where perverse legal and financial incentives have encouraged inappropriate over-treatment of patients of all ages. In the UK, the "vain pursuit of immortality" is a health economist's fantasy; it is not and never has been a feature of health services for older people here. Older people do not expect immortality and rarely fear death. What they want, and what the NHS tries to foster, are dignity and autonomy.

Williams' insistence that older people achieve less benefit from treatment than do the young is only true if one accepts his idea of what constitutes benefit. In terms of saving lives or quality of life older people may actually have more to gain than the young. Thrombolytic therapy in acute myocardial infarction[1] or beta-blockers afterwards[2] will save more lives per thousand patients treated if given to older people rather than younger. Ambulatory peritoneal dialysis for endstage renal failure provides a better quality of life for older patients than for younger.[3]

The output of health services (as distinct from public health measures) is not the prevalent health of the population but the changes in health status of individuals who use the services. The issue is how those changes should be valued. Williams's position is collectivist; what matters to him is the external value of the individual to the state. My view is that the valuation of outcomes should be that of the individuals seeking or receiving them. I derive this view from what I believe to be the values on which British society is based. Surely Williams would agree that "the values of the citizenry as a whole" must override the values of health economists as "a particular interest group"? It is also the individual and not the state who should decide when he or she has had a fair innings. (In the real world of

113

health care patients commonly tell their doctors and nurses when they are ready to return to the pavilion.) Williams attempts to equate our different views by implying that, because a younger person has longer to live, he will necessarily value his life more than an old person will value hers. This is clearly not necessarily true, and it does not solve the problem of the incommensurability of self evaluated lives. One commentator has suggested that the incommensurability problem could be overcome by the "willingness-to-pay" paradigm. This is illusory; it merely transfers the incommensurability from monadic valuations of living to monadic valuations of money.

Williams makes statements about average differences between young and old people, and implies that these differences will necessarily apply to individuals. It is true that on average older people are less fit or more susceptible to disease than the young, but there is wide individual variation. Many people in their 70s and 80s are functioning physiologically and psychologically in the normal range for people in their 20s and 30s. Some younger people are near the end of their natural life. People surely have a right to expect to be treated as individuals not as uniform members of a class, whether based on sex, skin colour, wealth, or age.

It is a depressing reflection on the human condition that most people use their rational minds not so much to decide what to do but rather to find plausible reasons for doing what they were going to do anyway. Prejudice against older people can be found in influential places in Britain, and rational argument alone may not be sufficient to protect them from cruelty and exploitation. People of some other nations seem to have kinder and more equitable attitudes towards their older fellow citizens.[4] It would be good to know why.

Older people are not defenceless. They represent over a quarter of the electorate, and if they can learn to vote tactically they have the power to unseat any government we are likely to labour under. In the USA, older people have used their voting power very effectively in improving their access to health care. It would be a pity if we have to go down that path as it inevitably raises the spectre of inter-generational conflict. There is surely something seriously wrong with a society where people cannot expect to have their rights defined and respected without having to wield some kind of threat.

I have been rebuked for suggesting that we might have less of a rationing problem if we spent a little more on health. I am unrepentant. We spend around £800 per person per year on health compared with £1400 in France and over £1600 in Germany. Perhaps we never could afford to spend enough entirely to avoid rationing, but it is worth considering that, if we spent a little more, we might be able to shift the rationing debate from questions of life and death to agonies over tattoo removal and breast

114

enhancement. Those are not trivial matters to the individuals concerned but they are a little more remote from basic rights.

1 ISIS-2 Collaborative Group. Randomised trial of intravenous streptokinase, oral aspirin, both, or neither among 17 187 cases of suspected myocardial infarction: ISIS-2. *Lancet* 1988;**ii**:349–60.
2 Hawkins CM, Richardson DW, Vokonas PS. Effect of propanolol in reducing mortality in older myocardial infarction patients. The beta-blocker heart attack trial experience. *Circulation* 1983;**67**(supp I):I-94–7.
3 Winnearls CG, Oliver DO, Auer J. Age and dialysis. *Lancet* 1992;**339**:432.
4 Nord E, Richardson J, Street A, Khuse H, Singer P. Maximising health benefits vs egalitarianism: an Australian survey of health issues. *Soc Sci Med* 1995;**41**:1429–37.

The case against

JOHN GRIMLEY EVANS

Older people are discriminated against in the NHS. This is best documented in substandard treatment of acute myocardial infarction and other forms of heart disease, where it leads to premature deaths and unnecessary disability. The care for older people with cancer is also poorer than that provided for younger patients.

Age discrimination in the NHS occurs despite explicit statements from the government that withholding treatment on the basis of age is not acceptable. Ageism is mostly instigated by clinicians but condoned by managers. Fundholding general practitioners have a financial incentive to deprive older patients of expensive healthcare, but there is no ready way to find out whether they do so. Whatever its full extent, the documented instances of age discrimination, together with the occasional published apologia for ageism, show that the morality of age based rationing should be a matter of public concern.

Need to assess individual risk

It is important to be clear what we are talking about. It is proper for a doctor to withhold treatment or investigation that is likely to do more harm than good to a patient. In an individual case actual outcome depends on the patient's physiological condition. The prevalence of impairments that shift the risk–benefit ratio adversely increases with age, so where individual physiological condition is used as the basis for allocating treatment older

115

people are more likely on average to be excluded than are younger people. Nevertheless, wide individual variation exists in ageing, and many people in later life function physiologically within the normal range for people much younger. The key issue, therefore, is that each decision should be made on a competent assessment of individual risk.

What I am objecting to is the exclusion from treatment on the basis of a patient's age without reference to his or her physiological condition. The patient is being treated as though he or she necessarily had properties identical with those corresponding to the average of the age group. We can draw a contrast with social class and skin colour. Should we withhold health care from members of lower social classes or from black people because of the poorer average outcome of their groups? Rather, most of us would suggest that extra attention should be paid to vulnerable members of such groups to try to compensate for their disadvantage. Why should old people not be viewed similarly?

Ethics, ideology, and the law

I am convinced that in the UK at present it is unethical to use age as a criterion for depriving people of health care from which they could benefit. The fundamental issue is ideological; and ideologies—and the ethical systems derived from them—can change with circumstances. The notion, implicit in the writings of many ethicists, that there is an objective basis for a universal ethical system is a dangerous illusion. Ethics are no more than logical deductions from primary ideologies. Ideologies are primary in the sense that they cannot be validated by any objective means. They can arise in various ways, and in England they arose by a long process of mutual adaptation of heterogeneous people developing efficient ways of living together. Not having a written constitution, we have in Britain to deduce the ideological principles of our society from our history and from the shared rhetoric of our major political parties.

From these I conclude that in times of peace British national values include the equality of citizens in their relation to the institutions of the state and acknowledgment of, and respect for, the uniqueness of individuals regardless of their physical or mental attributes. From the last follows the equal right of all citizens to live as they wish so long as they do not impede the like rights of others. If these ideas are indeed embodied in the ideology of British society, ageism, as well as racism and sexism, will be unethical.

The founts of ageism

Several factors generate or are invoked to justify ageism in health care.

Exploitation of the weak

The first is an issue of realpolitik. When healthcare managers aim to control costs older people are natural victims. They do not riot; they are uncomplaining and politically inactive. The threat of tactical voting by the militant elderly people of the USA caused a major shift in health and social care resources to their benefit. Although comprising more than a quarter of the electorate in Britain, old people are not yet seen by politicians as potential tactical voters. Inevitably they suffer, and inevitably ageism remains legal.

Professional ignorance

Ageism may arise from well intentioned ignorance, where health professionals assume incorrectly that older patients will be harmed rather than benefited by treatment. In reality the absolute benefit of some treatments—in terms, say, of deaths prevented—increases with prior risk whereas the probability of side effects remains constant. Where prior risk rises with age such treatments may be more effective given to older people than to younger. Moreover, except in the limited area of intensive care medicine, we still know little about the physiological variables that determine individual risks of benefit and harm from medical interventions. We need more research to enable meaningful negotiation over options for care with patients of all ages and to underpin more efficient targeting of resources.

Prejudice

The most important source of ageism is prejudice. Surveys in Britain show that older people are widely seen as of lower social worth than younger, but little has been done to explore the origins and dynamics of this prejudice. Some researchers suggest that public attitudes displayed by such surveys are a valid basis for rationing in the health services. There are several problems with this facile suggestion. People answering questions in a way that indicates low valuation of older people may do so not because of what they really feel but because of what they think the interviewer will regard as the "right" answer.

Typically, questions are in "doctor's dilemma" format in which there is treatment available for only one of two people who differ in age. The possibility of generating equity by allocating the treatment on the toss of a coin is not usually offered and is unlikely to be thought of spontaneously by the average citizen. It is also naive to assume that attitudes exposed by the desperate situation simulated in a doctor's dilemma would also emerge

117

in decisions on real life issues such as the relative lengths of waiting lists for hip replacements and hernia repairs.

Survey interviews are rarely confidential and do not contain control questions in which the two potential patients differ, say, in skin colour. Would researchers suggest that racial prejudice revealed by their questionnaires should be a basis for health service rationing? We may presume not; it would be recognised, as it should be for ageism, that the respondents were failing to conform to the principles of British society. To imply, as some have found it convenient to claim in the ageism debate, that it is paternalistic to esteem the values of society above the ignorant prejudices of some of its members is to confuse demagoguery with democracy.

The power of economics

Economists sometimes claim that their discipline is so fundamental that it can provide a sufficient basis for allocating society's resources in health care. Whether this assertion is acceptable or not is an ethical issue. It can be argued that economists should be restricted to identifying the most cost effective way of achieving a pattern of allocation that has been defined on ideological grounds. We have lived so long under a theocracy of markets, competition, and cost containment that people may forget that these are driven by an ideology of no more validity than the ideology behind common cause, collaboration, and social purpose that it supplanted.

Alan Williams has suggested that, if allocations of resources based on quality adjusted life years (QALYs) are thought to bear too heavily on older people, their needs can be weighted to conform more closely with externally derived principles of equity. This approach has the advantage of making the ethical input both explicit and manifestly the responsibility of those who provide it. Virtue still emerges wearing what many will see as the indecency of a price tag. Williams's dialectic derives from what he sees as a necessary trade off between equity and efficiency. In my view his notion of what should be regarded as efficiency in the NHS is questionable. We can find common ground in the assertion that healthcare resources should be allocated so as to do the most good. The ethical argument crystallises round what view of good should prevail.

There are two perspectives on a health service. On the one side are the purveyors, who, like shareholders in a chain of grocery shops, look for the best return on their investment. They may well think it appropriate to measure this return in terms of some measure such as QALYs gained. On the other are the users of the service. Although the NHS has in recent years been forced into a Procrustean bed of market imagery, the average British citizen sees it not as a chain of grocery shops but as something

118

more akin to a motoring organisation to which he pays a subscription so that it will be there to do what he wants when he wants it. He will judge the service on the extent to which it meets his informed desires. There is no reason to expect that maximising the production of QALYs will lead to the same recipe for distributing limited resources as maximising the achievement of users' informed wishes.

British citizens as taxpayers might see themselves alongside Williams with the purveyors, but as potential patients would, I suspect, ally themselves more consistently with the users. My assessment is that the users' perspective also provides a rationale more consonant with national values and with the explicit intentions for the NHS at its foundation. There are also unacceptable implications in the purveyors' approach.

First, measurement of output in units based on life years directly or indirectly puts different values on individuals according to their life expectancy. Thus citizens are no longer equal, and older people in particular are disadvantaged. Second, it assumes that the value of life, at any given level of objectively assessed disability, is determined by its length. But if we assert the unique individuality of citizens, the only person who can put a value on a life is the person living it. Lives of individuals are therefore formally incommensurable and it is mathematically as well as ethically improper to pile weighted valuations of them together as an aggregable commodity like tonnes of coal. There have been nations whose ideologies value citizens only for their potential collective usefulness to the state as soldiers, workers, or breeding females. In the UK, at least for the time being, are we not spirits of another sort?

The "fair innings" argument

This argument asserts that we have a right only to a certain number of years of life and after then only palliative as distinct from therapeutic care should be provided. Although sometimes mistaken for an economic argument, the fair innings approach will not necessarily save money unless we apply its corollary of compulsory euthanasia at the end of the innings. Palliative care can be more expensive than therapeutic care; the money saved by not providing coronary artery surgery for an elderly woman may be spent several times over if she has to live for months in a nursing home because of her angina.

The fair innings argument has historical roots in Christian theology and its requirement for time to earn one's place in heaven by purging the sins of youth with the good works of later life. For secular man fair innings now codes for two crucially different ideas which commentators sometimes confuse. The first is that as individuals we commonly come to a time when we conclude that we have done all that we wished and were able to do,

119

and that life no longer offers the potential of interest or pleasure that might make it preferable to oblivion. For some others of us death may at a particular time offer personal meaning, climactic consummation, or a perfected symbolism to our lives. Dying for a worthy cause may seem better than survival in servitude, failure, or dishonour. Such ideas underlie the existential concept of a fair innings or natural lifespan. Only the person living a life can say when it is complete in this sense, and its length for different individuals might range from 18 to 120 years.

The other version of a fair innings is that owing to overpopulation space on earth has to be rationed and after a time one should make way for someone else to enjoy life. (We could, of course, solve the underlying problem by controlling birth rates rather than limiting lifespan, but let us follow the logical trail.) This form of the fair innings is identified with a fixed number of years, usually assigned by Western authors to the high 70s. The assumption is that life confers some kind of intrinsic good that we can perhaps code as "happiness".

In its simplest form the argument requires that everyone has the same chance of happiness so that the fairness of the innings can be assessed by its length. Clearly this is not true. If the fairness of the innings is actually the area under a happiness/duration curve, the notion should lead to the early turning off of the rich and fortunate in favour of the poor and deprived. It would be theoretically possible to calculate an individual's fair innings allowance on the basis of some form of "happy life expectancy" adjusted for relevant variables such as social class and sex. Whether one should regard this as a serious possibility or an intellectually charming reductio ad absurdum depends on one's estimate of its potential utility. Given their longer life expectancy, women would probably have to take second place to men in access to health care. Rich older people would still, presumably, be able to purchase, in the private sector or abroad, treatments denied to them by the NHS. The fair innings concept is unlikely to provide an acceptable solution to problems of inequity.

Conclusion

Healthcare resources in Britain are limited, but only because the government limits them. If we continue with the healthcare budget restricted to some 7% of gross national product rationing is likely also to continue. In a democratic society rationing should be explicit and transparently the responsibility of government. For several reasons it would be timely for Britain to define what its national values and the rights and duties of its citizens are. I should be disturbed if these turned out to differ essentially from those deduced above. If these values are to be translated into the NHS, primary rationing has to focus on equitable limits to the type and volume of services. We should not create, on the basis of age or any other characteristic over which individuals have no control, classes of Untermenschen whose lives and wellbeing are deemed not worth spending money on.

A rejoinder to John Grimley Evans

ALAN WILLIAMS

Coincidentally, at about the same time as the original pair of articles on this subject were published, there appeared two short reports which together highlighted perfectly the problem of fairness between the generations. One was from Age Concern, documenting widespread age based rationing in the NHS, and arguing that it was wrong and should cease. The other was from the Child Poverty Action Group, claiming that there were now more children living in poverty than pensioners living in poverty, and this was having a serious effect upon these children's health prospects, and should be remedied. So assuming that spending an extra £100m would have an equal effect on the health of both groups, who do you think should have priority? This is the question that has to be addressed.

I have no doubt that most doctors do take a patient's age into account when determining which treatment to offer (and not all such age discrimination is to the disadvantage of elderly people). Most doctors are caring and responsible people, so one should not assume that such age discrimination is arbitrary and capricious and ill-informed. If it were, there would be no justification for it whatever. If it is not, we should ask ourselves what possible justification could there be for it. That was, and is, my starting point.

It seems to me that there are two possible justifications. The first is that the benefits to be gained from a treatment may vary according to a person's age, and because one of the objectives of medicine is to be as beneficial as possible, age will influence which treatments are offered to which people. If older people have higher risks of complications, and are less likely to make a proper recovery from treatment, surely that is not something to be ignored? This kind of age discrimination is often defended by people on the grounds that it is "purely clinical" (and therefore exempt from moral scrutiny?). For them the real problem is when social conditions associated with ageing (for example, family support and housing situation) are taken

121

into account. Doctors frequently assert the significance of such social factors when they are making admission and discharge decisions for older people, so the notion of what is "purely clinical" seems rather flexible. And perhaps it should be. But it still requires discussion and justification. And I see no reason why, on moral grounds, it should not survive such scrutiny.

The second possible justification is rather more problematic, because it depends crucially on whether you think that one of the objectives of the NHS is to reduce inequalities in people's experience of health over their lifetime. I believe this to have been one of the strongest motives of the founders of the NHS, and therefore something that deserves to be given some weight. But even if you personally do not subscribe to it, you cannot argue that it is an intrinsically immoral principle, and therefore incapable of providing justification for age discrimination by those who do believe that it is a proper objective for the NHS to pursue. It is this objective that generates the "fair innings" argument, not in the extreme form set out by Grimley Evans in his original companion piece to mine, but in the more moderate form in which I set it out. In essence, it says that those who have had better than average health over their entire lifetime should accept rather less being done for them than will be done to improve the prospects of those who will otherwise finish up below average. In health terms, the haves should help the have nots. This does not mean that the haves get nothing. With progressive income taxes (which are designed to help redistribute income from the haves to the have nots), we do not impose 100% marginal tax rates on anybody, but we do impose higher marginal tax rates on the rich (the haves) than on the poor (the have nots), and this is widely regarded as the fairest of all taxes. Similarly, with health care, we should be prepared to spend rather more to provide a given level of benefit for a have not than for a have. And in health terms the "haves" are people who have reached a good age with a good health record, and the "have nots" are the younger people (which in this context includes the middle aged!) who have little prospect of enjoying a healthy old age. That is what the "fair innings" argument is all about. And, whether you agree with it or not, it seems to me to provide a perfectly respectable moral argument in favour of taking age into account (among other things) when setting priorities for health care. It gives more weight to the position of the Child Poverty Action Group than to the arguments of Age Concern.

Various correspondents responding to the rather garbled accounts of my argument which appeared in the popular press have put forward a counter argument, which I had not considered earlier, and which I must now consider. It is that the people who are now over 70 are those who suffered great hardships in the war, and therefore deserve our special sympathy. The implication is that whatever may be the case with future generations of elderly people, the current generation should be an exception. I think that this argument carries little weight in the context of health care.

122

Obviously, those whose health is adversely affected by war (or by other experiences of public service, at whatever age) are entitled to such health care as is available to deal with those health problems. We may even decide that those whose health was adversely affected by public service deserve more than those whose health was adversely affected in other ways. But this is quite different from a broad based argument that everyone who was born between certain selected years is entitled to special treatment (whether the war adversely affected their health or not). Today's fit 80 year olds may well have been favourably affected (in health terms) by the war, because it has been well established that through food rationing the health of many poorer people was greatly improved. The war was not bad for everybody's health. Perhaps we can help today's poor children to have a healthier future by the more equitable rationing of health care without relying on a war to do it for us.

9 Central government should have a greater role in rationing decisions

The political and administrative centre should have an increased role in making healthcare rationing decisions

The case for

JO LENAGHAN

Rationing decisions in the NHS have largely been controlled by the medical profession and have tended to be implicit, with little reference to agreed systems or criteria.[1] Central government is responsible for deciding how resources for health care are distributed around Britain and sets the legal context, but should it do more and develop a national framework for rationing health care? A recent spate of reports and articles revealing variations in the provision of and access to healthcare services highlights the urgent need to address this question.

The House of Commons Select Committee on Health surveyed the priority setting practices of 49 health authorities, noting: "We have been struck by the seemingly enormous variation in access across the country."[2] Redmayne revealed that one in six health authorities are now excluding treatments from public provision,[3] whereas a recent survey has shown that couples in Scotland are seven times more likely to get NHS in vitro fertilisation than those in the south west region.[4]

Variations in healthcare provision are nothing new, but the purchaser–provider split has made them more explicit, and, more importantly, revealed variations in the criteria used to justify these decisions. For example, in Humberside fertility treatment is provided to women until the age of 40, whereas Liverpool provides it until the age of 35.[2] As New and Le Grand have observed, explicit rationing has not been accompanied by an explicit or shared understanding on how such decisions should be made.[1]

It has been argued that, if the government increased the amount of resources available to the NHS, then this would remove the need to ration.

124

However, this ignores the fact that decisions about whether to provide a treatment are not always determined by financial considerations alone. For instance, the new genetic technologies may cause us to question not just whether we can afford to fund particular types of screening but also whether it is appropriate for the NHS to provide certain services at all.[5] Such issues raise fundamental questions about the nature and purpose of our health service, the rights of citizens, and the responsibilities of professionals, and are too important to be left to individual health authorities and medical practitioners to resolve alone.

Lack of coherence

From April 1996 each health authority has had an explicit and different working definition of health care (funded by the NHS) and social care (means tested). Definitions of what constitutes a terminal illness, and therefore qualifies for NHS funded palliative care, vary between health authorities, from 2 weeks' to 12 months' life expectancy.[6] This unacceptable variation not only causes problems for the individuals concerned but also helps to fuel public fears. What and who is the NHS for? What is an illness? What treatments can we legitimately be expected to receive on the NHS, to which all citizens contribute?

Doctors and health authorities have responded to increased demand and reduced budgets by limiting or delaying the services they provide. This not only makes life difficult for those involved in providing and planning health services, but as the process becomes more transparent it also increases the anxiety and uncertainty of those who use the NHS. Some have argued that rationing decisions, to be responsive and flexible, must be left to the micro level. Rationing, they claim, is essentially a messy business.[7] However, as Kennedy has written, this "ad hocery" means that medical practice lacks an internal coherence and consistency of principle, and therefore the interests of patients, doctors, and the community are not fully served.[8] The challenge is surely to identify what kind of decisions can be taken appropriately at the micro, meso, and macro levels.

Erosion of public confidence

The lack of a coherent vision of what and who the NHS is for is in danger of undermining public confidence. The increased media interest in issues such as Child B and the withdrawal of NHS provision of long term care has helped fuel anxiety among the public, who fear that the NHS will no longer provide a comprehensive service, free at the point of delivery.[9]

Some critics have argued that the creation of an explicit policy on rationing will erode public confidence. This position fails to acknowledge that public confidence is already ebbing. The Institute for Public Policy Research pilot citizens' juries have suggested that the more information you give people, the more confidence they have in the NHS.[10] If left unchecked, health authorities are bound to continue to exclude various treatments. The media and the opposition parties are well aware of the publicity to be gained from such incidents, and the public will be left confused. The private sector is likely to benefit from this increasing uncertainty.

Equity and local flexibility

Inequity of access may have been an unwanted occurrence in the NHS of the past, but it now appears to be built into the current system.[11] The logic of the internal market and the devolving of powers to individual health authorities have made geographical variations in provision of healthcare services not just more common, but inevitable. As argued above, however, it is not just the variations themselves which give cause for concern, but the variations in the criteria used to make such decisions.

In the case of in vitro fertilisation, for example, it is often non-needs based characteristics which can determine whether a woman gains access to treatment. A decision may depend on where she lives, whether she is married, or how old she is, and these criteria vary from region to region. The variations in provision reveal that we do not have equal rights to treatment and care and that finite resources for health care are being distributed according to criteria not solely based on clinical judgment.

The goal of equality is increasingly being sacrificed to the new religion of "local flexibility". This is indeed an important aim, but, as New and Le Grand have argued, the level of service may reasonably vary according to geography, but whether a service should be provided or not should not vary between regions as this may offend our sense of territorial justice.[1]

Others have argued that the responsibility for purchasing health care should lie with local authorities.[12] This idea certainly has merit, and the Institute for Public Policy Research has argued that this should be piloted.[13] Nevertheless, as New has pointed out, "this might cause difficulties for a national health strategy, geographic equity and allocating between finance between 'free' health care and means tested social care".[14]

Competence and legitimacy

The House of Commons Select Committee on Health expressed its concern at the variations in competence between different health authorities.[2] The members of health authorities are appointed by the Secretary of State, and as such are not elected or accountable to the public. Rationing decisions are political decisions, as they involve the distribution of public money. These quangos seem to lack both the competence and the legitimacy to make rationing decisions on our behalf.

It is perhaps tempting at this point to retort "leave it to the doctors", but do doctors possess any more legitimacy or competence for rationing decisions than health authorities? Kennedy has argued that the issue of whether a treatment is effective or not is clearly a medical decision, but whether or not a treatment is the best use of public funds is a political decision.[8] Other issues, such as quality of life, involve questions of moral and ethical concern. All of these are involved in a medical decision, but are beyond the competence and legitimacy of a doctor to resolve alone. The medical profession has recognised this for some time and has called on the government to share the burden of these difficult decisions. Converting political problems into medical problems[15] might be convenient for politicians, but it overburdens doctors, excludes the public from debate, and prevents us from holding the decision makers to account.

Others have expressed concern at the prospect of local authorities purchasing health care, for fear that this will "legitimise" unpopular or unfair rationing decisions. Indeed, will the public perceive regional variations in healthcare provision to be legitimate if made by elected bodies? New and Le Grand warn of a "legitimisation crisis" if the NHS is unable to distribute resources fairly or match expectations.[1] As Busse et al have observed, for the benefits provided through the welfare system to provide solidarity they must be comprehensive enough for the recipients to value them and provide a clear element of redistribution in order for the nation to appreciate the solidarity.[16]

To argue for a greater role for the centre in rationing decisions does not mean that there will be no room for local flexibility. Indeed a code of practice, developed at the centre, could provide a framework within which local decision making could flourish. The challenge is to develop a policy which enables us to define the limits and extent of local flexibility, rather than allowing it to continue to be used as an excuse for all manner of inappropriate variations.

A greater role for the centre

To increase the coherence and legitimacy of decision making in the NHS, we need to redefine what kind of decisions are appropriate to be taken at which level. We need to define the boundaries within which doctors can be free to exercise their clinical judgment, and create a principled framework within which health authorities and managers can legitimately make their decisions.

The Institute for Public Policy Research has rejected the idea of a defined package of care and instead has proposed a national advisory body to develop appropriate national guidelines, within which the different groups can exercise their particular skills and judgment.[9] A national health commission should be set up to advise parliament on devising guidelines and a code of practice. This would draw on a wide range of experience and skill, involving all interested parties in the process and pooling ideas. Its aim would be to build a broad consensus for the criteria by which decisions about resource allocation for health care can reasonably be made and to keep matters under review. Our recommendations are similar to proposals made by the Royal College of Physicians[17] and are consistent with the findings of a pilot citizens' jury on rationing.[18] Our proposals are based on an assessment of the experience of other countries, which suggests that rationing by exclusion is neither helpful nor desirable and that developing guidelines in order to ensure fair and consistent decision making processes offers a pragmatic way forward.[9,19,20] The exact mechanisms and functions of the proposed commission are discussed in detail in the report, *Rationing and rights in health care.*[9]

Although at the end of the day doctors must actually take the decisions in the surgery, the clinic, and the ward, the criteria they use should conform to standards which are seen to be consensual, legitimate, and consistently applied. More open and fair decisions will help to rebuild public trust and establish new relationships between all the stakeholders.

Possible objections

It has been suggested that any attempt at rational rationing is futile and that it would be impossible for any national body to reach a consensus on the difficult issues it would be asked to resolve. If rationing issues are too difficult to resolve on a national level, involving all the expert and interest groups, then what chance do hard pushed local health authorities have? Surely the recognition that rationing is so difficult merely demonstrates the need for us to pool our knowledge and experiences? Rationing, of course, neither can and never should be reduced to a precise mathematical formula, but it should be possible to develop rationing policies that are socially acceptable and which conform to standards of common justice.

Other complaints, such as increasing bureaucracy and costs, limiting clinical freedom, etc, all depend on what kind of policies are created, and with what objectives. They also depend on the level of public involvement and support, and on how much professional confidence such policies can command. None of these legitimate concerns should be dismissed lightly, but potential problems can be overcome by commitment and imagination, and cannot justify inaction. Once we have agreed that the centre does need to have a greater role in rationing decisions, we can then begin to debate the form which such a policy should take, in order to ensure that these concerns are fully addressed.

As New has argued, views about rationing may remain persistently polarised among members in society, thereby increasing the need to develop democratic systems of decision making in order to resolve these conflicts. It is unlikely that different views will ever be entirely reconciled, but it should be possible to build confidence and support for the process by which such decisions are made.[14]

Conclusion

The arguments in favour of a greater role for the centre in rationing decisions must be compared not to some imaginary perfect future but to the poverty of the status quo. New policies always involve risks, but the option of doing nothing is far from risk free. If we fail to tackle rationing in the NHS, if we leave the health authorities to muddle through, the media to seize on the inevitable inequities, and the public to worry about the consequences, then the middle classes may increasingly turn to private insurance in pursuit of peace of mind, eventually reducing the NHS to a safety net service for the poor.

We have a clear choice: either we attempt to shape the future of the future of healthcare provision in the public interest, or we allow it to be shaped for us, by the workings of the internal market, the influence of vested interests, and the ad hoc decisions of individual health authorities. The future of the health service in the UK is too important to be shaped by default. For the NHS to survive and succeed in the next century it must earn the trust of the public, and therefore it must offer services which all citizens value, and allocate its resources in a manner which is seen to be fair. A greater role for the centre in rationing health care may help us to achieve these aims.

1 New B, Le Grand J. *Rationing in the NHS: principles and pragmatism*. London: King's Fund, 1996.
2 House of Commons Health Committee. *Priority setting in the NHS: purchasing*, Vol 1. Annex 1. London: HMSO, 1995.
3 Redmayne S. *Reshaping the NHS: strategies and priorities amid resource allocation*. Birmingham: NAHAT, 1995:51.
4 *Report of fourth national survey of NHS funding of infertility services*. London: National Institute for Assisted Conception, 1995.
5 McLean SMA. Mapping the human genome: friend or foe. *Soc Sci Med* 1996;**39**:1221–7.
6 Marwick S. *Eligibility criteria for continuing health care: palliative care*. London: National Council for Hospice and Specialist Palliative Care Services, 1996.
7 Hunter DJ. Rationing health care: the political perspective. *Br Med Bull* 1995;**51**:876–84.

8 Kennedy I. What is a medical decision? In: Kennedy I, ed. *Treat me right: essays in medical law and ethics*. Oxford: Clarendon Press, 1988.

9 Lenaghan J. *Rationing and rights in health care*. London: IPPR, 1996.

10 Coote A, Lenaghan J. *Citizens' juries. Theory into practice*. London: IPPR, 1997.

11 Dickson N. Blood sweat and tears. *Guardian* 1996; 16 Sep.

12 Harrison S. Hunter DJ, Johnston IH, Nicholson N, Thurnhurst C, Wistow G. *Health before health care*. London: IPPR, 1991.

13 Cooper L, Coote A, Davies A, Jackson C. *Voices off*. London: IPPR, 1995.

14 New B on behalf of the Rationing Agenda Group. The rationing agenda in the NHS. *BMJ* 1996;312:1593–601.

15 Klein R. *The new politics of the NHS*. 3rd ed. London: Longman, 1995:23.

16 Busse R, Howorth C, Schwartz FW. The future development of the rights-based approach to health care in Germany: more rights or fewer? In Lenaghan J, ed. *Hard choices in health care*. London: BMJ Publishing Group, 1996.

17 Royal College of Physicians. *Setting priorities in the NHS: a framework for decision making*. London: RCP, 1995.

18 Lenaghan J, New B, Mitchell E. Setting priorities: is there a role for citizens' juries? *BMJ* 1996;312:1591–3.

19 Ham C. Health care rationing. *BMJ* 1995;310:1483–4.

20 McKee M, Figueras J. Setting priorities: can Britain learn from Sweden? *BMJ* 1996;312: 691–4.

A rejoinder to Jo Lenaghan

STEPHEN HARRISON

There is more in common than of difference between Lenaghan's position and my own. We both agree that the present NHS quangos lack the legitimacy to undertake rationing, which is a true political decision. We agree that, although clinical autonomy is desirable and necessary, there are limits as to what should be left to it, and that what is not left to it should be explicit rather than implicit. She is rightly concerned that the apparently arbitrary differences between health authorities fuel public concerns and undermine confidence in the NHS. Indeed, there is nothing incoherent about Lenaghan's arguments; it is simply that they can lead to other conclusions in addition to her own.

Although it is true that inequity of access is apparent within the present system, it is not clear that these inequities extend beyond specific services or interventions. Indeed, to the extent that the NHS capitation (allocation) formula is equitable, and on the assumption that NHS institutions have roughly the same level of efficiency, then a crude overall equity of service provision must exist. Lenaghan is correct to point to the experience of citizens' juries: information (and, she might have added, deliberation) increases public confidence.

130

What follows is that a revised arrangement for healthcare rationing should meet two criteria. First, the public should have more information about healthcare interventions, and about the local uses of healthcare resources in comparison to other localities. Second, the criteria that underpin rationing decisions should be transparent. These considerations can apply as well to my proposals for local government authorities as to Lenaghan's proposals for a national body to advise health authorities. Indeed we both propose some central involvement: in my case legislation to preclude rationing on the basis of social judgments, and to require the general pursuit of equity of outcome. We also both propose some local difference.

What appears to divide my position from Lenaghan's is my rejection of any coherent role for NHS quangos, whose continuing existence she implicitly endorses. It is, of course, true that social solidarity requires a reasonably comprehensive core of services, but there is no reason to imagine that local authority purchasers of NHS services would, for instance, massively reduce acute general medical services in favour of expenditure on some untried technology or on elective cosmetic surgery.

The case against

STEPHEN HARRISON

As components of democracy, the health authorities currently responsible for the local governance of the NHS are a nonsense. As Regan and Stewart pointed out 15 years ago,[1] their quasi-independent statutory existence precludes clear accountability on the part of the political centre yet without (as in the old nationalised industries) providing a clearly delegated management role, and without providing local democratic accountability. Health authorities, especially given recent suspicions surrounding the closed nature of the appointments process, are truly examples of Stewart's "new magistracy":[2] unelected, unaccountable, and tacitly assumed to refrain from challenging the status quo.

The rationing of health care is inevitable in any system of third party payment for health care,[3,4] and where the system is publicly or quasi-publicly financed rationing decisions are political decisions in the sense both of requiring accountability for public funds and of involving the allocation of resources which may significantly affect people's life chances. This remains so whether or not they are taken on party political lines and

131

whether or not they involve substantial technical input (about, for instance, the efficacy of specific healthcare interventions).

It follows that health authorities are not appropriate bodies to be making such decisions. As Regan and Stewart noted more generally, the consequences of the present arrangements are threefold.[1] First, the centralisation of electoral accountability means that in practice there is none. The centre does not have "the time or resources to provide more than partial, selective and spasmodic accountability". Second, the attempt even to provide that much leads to administrative and political congestion. Third, these arrangements leave a highly unsatisfactory role for the people who are appointed as authority members. If all this is so, reform in relation to healthcare rationing might logically take one of two directions.

A stronger role for the centre?

One is to posit an increased role for the centre. There are strong temptations to opt for such a solution, especially when faced with the difficult questions that can arise in relation to healthcare rationing. After all, the UK is a small country with predominantly national news media with a strong tendency to report regional differences in public provision as problematic by definition. This increasingly national focus on politics has been enthusiastically reinforced by government policy—for example, through its use of performance indicators in health and education, and its erosion of local democracy by reducing local authority functions and autonomy (for instance by capping local taxes). In the specific case of the NHS the use of the term "national" provides ready rhetoric against the development or even continuation of local diversity. Not surprisingly, therefore, the appearance of painful local political questions about how to ration health care leads to calls for the political and administrative centre to take an enhanced role.

Such a central approach to healthcare rationing is not indefensible, and various schemes have been proposed. These range from the enactment of procedural rights as proposed by Lenaghan[5] to the development of a national package of permitted treatments for specified clinical conditions, defined either in terms of some rough cost–utility criteria (as in the Oregon formula) or by some other criterion such as Dworkin's prudent insurance principle.[6]

A pragmatic proposition

However, such approaches are not the only practicable solution and I want to show that the alternative approach is feasible: increased involvement

132

for the political and administrative locality. In so arguing, I make what is essentially a pragmatic proposition, based on the possibility of adapting an existing institution, local government, to perform a rationing function in health care in a way which conforms to some principles which I presume to be widely held (democracy and transparent accountability) and which offers an enhanced opportunity for the pursuit of equity of health outcome, an objective which may not be so widely approved.

I need to set out some preliminary points. First, nothing in this essay is intended to undermine the present role of the political centre in the geographical allocation of resources for the NHS through the capitation formula or some improvement in it. Indeed, such an arrangement is a crucial underpinning of the proposal. Second, nothing in this essay is intended to diminish the case for public services to be the subject of consultation with their users[7]; although I am concerned here with public participation in a broader sense, user consultation remains an important component.

Third, this essay is about the explicit rationing of health care. Of course defensible cases for implicit rationing exist,[8-10] and it is also possible to infer from opinion poll data a public preference for rationing to be effected implicitly through clinical decisions.[11,12] However, adherents to such a position do not argue for an increased central role (either procedural or substantive) since such a role itself implies explicitness, and the terms of the particular debate to which this essay is a contribution therefore exclude consideration of the general merits of explicitness. I would add, though, that implicitness precludes the possibilities of democracy and transparency.

Fourth, I do not subscribe to the view that healthcare rationing can be neatly divided into questions of what treatments are to be available and of which patients are to receive these treatments. One reason for this is that while British clinicians have substantial autonomy in relation to the latter (and my own opinion is that this is desirable) such autonomy is not inevitable, as anyone who has observed the managed care practices of US health insurers will be aware. The other, more important, reason is that treatment and patient are logically inseparable in the context of rationing (the Oregon formula employed treatment-condition pairs). It is not a question of deciding that treatment T is available, but of deciding that it is available for diagnosis X, the latter term perhaps including some assessment of severity. An obvious example is antibiotics; no one would argue that the NHS should not provide these at all, but a case could be made for withholding them from patients whose immune systems could be expected quickly to overcome the infection unaided. In other words, rationing cannot entirely be separated from clinical thresholds even though clinicians may be able to manipulate these.

Finally, the case that I am seeking to advance is a general one in favour of a greater local political role in NHS rationing, rather than a detailed organisational prescription. I have therefore not considered such practicalities as current local government reorganisation, the deprivation factors to be included in the capitation formula, or the structure and ownership of NHS trusts.

Local authorities as healthcare purchasers

Though local authorities had a substantial role in the provision of health care before 1948, the first post-NHS proposal for them to run the service was made by Regan and Stewart in 1982.[1] Revived in the subsequent context of the purchaser–provider split by Harrison et al,[6] it has also been supported by the Association of Metropolitan Authorities.[13] Essentially, the proposal is for local authorities to become responsible for the purchasing, and therefore the rationing, of health care for their resident populations. Care would continue to be provided by NHS trusts (which might themselves need to be democratised) and occasionally by the private sector. This proposal is underpinned by both a logic of democracy (with which this essay is mainly concerned) and a logic of equity.

The logic of democracy

A service which aims to serve a local community must be responsive to both the needs of that community and local values and priorities; indeed, these are hardly separable from each other. Despite current political rhetoric which claims that local political decision making has been superseded by a market which responds to individuals' needs, this is not so. As Bogdanor points out, the market in public services is an artificial one, created and regulated by government;[14] it cannot therefore be defended as if it were the impersonal outcome of individuals' interactions, and the NHS must do more than just respond to the preferences of its "consumers". It follows that local differences in priorities and provision should occur.

Elected local government provides a means of taking rationing decisions which are democratically legitimate, especially when accompanied by other mechanisms to enhance accountability, such as consultation with the public and user groups. In this way local differences will almost certainly occur; for instance, some might choose to establish specific healthcare rights for local residents, while others might prefer to establish broader objectives and to use waiting lists and clinical priority as a means of dispensing rough justice.[15] These differences should not be seen as a political problem provided that two conditions are met.

The first condition is that such differences can be legitimised, and the fact of local election provides one key element in such legitimisation and

134

hence the basis for independent action. Local authorities already have experience of explicit rationing both in the sense of deciding what needs to meet and of determining priorities between individuals; housing points systems and social care needs are obvious examples. As Hunter has noted, however, this is not a sufficient condition of legitimacy, but needs to be supplemented by ongoing consultation with the local public,[16] perhaps by such discursive means as citizens' juries[17] or by more reactive means such as the "talkback panel" shared by local and health authorities in Calderdale and Kirklees in west Yorkshire. It needs also to be supplemented by consultation with service user groups. The role of local government in the political life of the UK has been steadily undermined over the last two decades; to give it responsibility for purchasing health services would potentially offer a boost to popular perceptions of its importance.

The second condition is that resources are seen to be distributed and used equitably. There are several strands to this, in each of which the political centre does have a role.

First, NHS resources must be equitably distributed between local authorities, so that local differences are differences only of priority, rather than differences in total resource relative to need. If this is achieved, what may be called "healthcare migration" (that is individuals moving to an area where their treatment is a priority, rather as they might currently seek the schools that they prefer for their children) would not be a problem since a particular set of priorities would necessarily imply a set of non-priorities. Such equity might be achieved either by central distribution of resources along the lines of the present capitation formula or (in the unlikely event of a radical extension of local taxation powers) by a centrally determined needs adjustment factor.

Second, there should be no use of purely social judgments (about lifestyle, for instance) in establishing entitlement to services or treatments; as Doyal and Gough have noted, people have an ongoing need for health even if they have genuinely contributed to their present ill health.[18] This requirement not to discriminate might be the subject of legislation. Third, local authorities should be encouraged, again perhaps via legislation, to use their control over a range of health related policy areas (rather than just health services) to pursue broad equity of health outcome in such terms as life expectancy, disability, and longstanding illness. It seems unlikely that detailed legislation is appropriate for this; rather, a general statutory duty might be established, to be used as an audit criterion in Audit Commission evaluations of local authorities. The policy means by which authorities might pursue such equity are briefly discussed in the next section.

Suggestions, such as that made above, for the NHS to be democratised via local government have tended to produce rather contradictory criticisms, often from the same sources. Thus local government is typically portrayed as being not really democratic at all, but as both overbureaucratised

135

and overpoliticised, with important decisions made by councillors and a correspondingly reduced role for managers.[19] Leaving aside the dubious inference that British central government is a paragon of democracy, it is hard to see in them much other than a generalised hostility to local government. The scheme proposed above would help to relegitimise and reinvigorate local government.

The logic of equity

A key pragmatic advantage of local authority responsibility for health service purchasing would be the latter's co-location with policy responsibility for other local services which affect health. The most obvious examples are social services, public housing, environmental health, and local planning of roads and buildings. Such co-location would permit an integrated policy approach to health in place of the present rather artificial arrangement whereby health and health services are often treated as synonymous. Integrated policies would not, of course, be guaranteed,[20] though the proposal for a statutory duty to pursue equity of health outcome ought to provide an important incentive.

Unlike the arguments for local democracy, the arguments for local integration have had a good press.[21] However, recent central government policies which have had the effect of extending the means testing of social care pose an obvious difficulty for a fully integrated local health and social care service. To achieve such a service means that either means testing must be extended to health care, or abolished; neither seems politically feasible at present. Nevertheless, the responsibility of a single organisation for both services should help to undermine some of the incentives for cost shifting that currently exist.

Concluding remarks

My main purpose has been to argue that increasing the role of central government in healthcare rationing is not the only approach to tackling the present somewhat chaotic situation. Increasing the role of local government in a way which is underpinned by strategic, centrally determined rules is a feasible, and indeed preferable, alternative which should not simply be rubbished because it encounters long held prejudices of interested parties. The transfer to local government of the purchasing of health care offers a democratic input to its rationing and the possibility of a more integrated approach to health policy, enabling what I have called the logics of democracy and of equity to be reconciled.

1 Regan DE, Stewart J. An essay in the local government of health: the case for local authority control. *Social Policy and Administration* 1982;**16**:19–43.
2 Stewart JD. *Accountability to the public.* London: European Policy Forum, 1992.
3 Donaldson C, Gerard K. *Economics of health care financing: the visible hand.* London: Macmillan, 1993.
4 Harrison S, Hunter DJ. *Rationing health care.* London: Institute for Public Policy Research, 1994.
5 Lenaghan J. *Rationing and rights in health care.* London: Institute for Public Policy Research, 1996.
6 Harrison S, Hunter DJ, Johnston IH, Nicholson N, Thurnhurst C, Wistow G. *Health before health care.* London: Institute for Public Policy Research, 1991.
7 Knox C, McAlister D. Policy evaluation: incorporating users' views. *Public Administration* 1995;**73**:413–36.
8 Mechanic ,D. Professional judgment and the rationing of medical care. *University of Pennsylvania Law Review* 1992;**140**:1713–54.
9 Hoffenberg R. Rationing. *BMJ* 1992;**304**:182.
10 Hunter DJ. Rationing and health gain. *Critical Public Health* 1993;**4**:27–32.
11 Heginbotham C. Health care priority setting: a survey of doctors, managers and the general public. In: *Rationing in action.* London, BMJ Publishing Group, 1993.
12 Bowling A. Health care rationing: the public's debate. *BMJ* 1996;**312**:670–4.
13 Association of Metropolitan Authorities. *Local authorities and health services: a future role for local authorities in the purchasing of health services: a scoping paper.* London: AMA, 1993.
14 Bogdanor V. Local voices cry out in the quango wilderness. *Observer* 1994;20 Mar:4.
15 Boyd KM, ed. *The ethics of resource allocation in health care.* Edinburgh: University of Edinburgh Press, 1979.
16 Hunter DJ. The case for closer co-operation between local authorities and the NHS. *BMJ* 1995;**310**:587–9.
17 Stewart J, Kendall E, Coote A. *Citizens' juries.* London: Institute for Public Policy Research, 1994.
18 Doyal L, Gough I. *A theory of human need.* Basingstoke: Macmillan, 1991.
19 National Association of Health Authorities and Trusts. *Securing effective public accountability in the NHS: a discussion paper.* Birmingham: NAHAT, 1993.
20 Mays N. What are the effects of integration in the NI health and personal social services? *Critical Public Health* 1993;**4**:43–8.
21 Editorial. *Financial Times* 1991; 6 Jun.

A rejoinder to Stephen Harrison

JO LENAGHAN

Harrison correctly argues that increasing the role of government in healthcare rationing is not the only approach to tackling the present somewhat chaotic state of affairs. We both identify similar problems, agreeing that rationing is inevitable, that rationing decisions are political decisions, and that therefore it is not appropriate to leave health authorities to tackle these matters alone. Harrison is concerned with "the logic of democracy", and it is this that leads him to propose that local authorities

137

should become responsible for the purchasing and therefore the rationing of health care for their resident populations.

I agree that there is a strong case for devolving the purchasing function to local authorities and would support this proposal on democratic, as well as public health, grounds. However, I disagree with Harrison's claim that local authorities should also be responsible for rationing decisions and would suggest that such a reform would require a greater, rather than a lesser, role for the centre. Harrison suggests that because local authorities are elected "differences can be legitimised". This may be true at a technical level, but public perception may differ. There is increasing public disquiet about the variations in provision of long term care services and I doubt whether the recent decision by Birmingham Health Authority to end funding for fertility treatment would have been greeted with any less controversy had this decision been taken by elected councillors.

Harrison's proposals, although perhaps possessing greater logic and consistency than my own, fail to take account of the special space that the NHS occupies in the popular and political imagination; the notion of citizenship and entitlement; and the difference between perceived as opposed to technical legitimacy.

Harrison argues that local authorities have a duty to serve their local communities, responding to their needs, values, and priorities—but what of the wider community? What rights of access to public services do we share as a result of our citizenship of the UK, rather than the temporary rights arising from residence in a particular region of the country? The NHS is funded by national taxation, allowing governments to distribute fairly. On a sociopolitical level, this provides a rare and valuable opportunity for social solidarity to operate in practice. Policies that localise rationing problems may lead us to focus on what divides us rather than what unites us. On a more technical level, exactly what "values" in the context of healthcare rationing are likely to differ significantly between, say, Birmingham and Glasgow? There may be more differences (age, sex, religion, race, class, etc) within our cities than between them. The objective of a government should be to attempt to build consensus and support for a shared set of values which allow public services to be distributed in a way that is seen and understood to be fair and legitimate.

I therefore conclude that even if, as Stephen Harrison rightly suggests, local authorities are given responsibility for purchasing health care, this strengthens rather than weakens the argument for a greater role for the centre in rationing decisions. We need to establish the appropriate limits to local flexibility and clinical judgment within which local/health authorities and NHS professionals can legitimately operate.

10 Rationing within the NHS should be explicit

Rationing should be made explicit at all levels of NHS decision making

The case for

LEN DOYAL

Much recent discussion has revolved around whether the rationing of health care that is occurring within the NHS should be explicit or implicit.[1] Many commentators argue in favour of implicit rationing, for a range of reasons. Opinion appears to be divided between those who claim that implicit rationing will (1) be inevitable since there are no clear criteria on which to base explicit rationing, (2) make patients and providers happier, and (3) make the administrative and political processes of healthcare provision run more smoothly. I provide reasons for rejecting each of these contentions, arguing instead that explicit rationing is vital for the moral management of health care.

The argument from confused criteria

The creation of an internal market in the NHS appeared to place explicit rationing on the agenda of healthcare providers. Rationing had always occurred within the service but previously it had been camouflaged under clinical judgment. Now purchasers were to draw up plans showing how much was to be allocated to what type of care and why. Providers were to audit clinical staff to ensure that their work conformed to agreed criteria of effectiveness and all was to be open to public scrutiny.

The expected transparency has not occurred. Health authorities have generally not come clean about their inability to meet demand and have awarded block contracts primarily on the basis of past expenditure, with shortfalls shared between existing clinical services. As a result, the realities of rationing within the NHS have remained where they always were—with clinicians making decisions on the basis of varied and conflicting criteria, often dressed in the guise of clinical necessity.[2]

139

These developments have led to a weary resignation that any ambition to make rationing explicit within the NHS is hopelessly optimistic. It is argued that there are no clear rules according to which rationing should occur and a lack of political will to implement what criteria there are. For example, the health committee of the House of Commons proclaims: "There is no such thing as a correct set of priorities, or even a correct way of setting priorities."[3] Klein concurs: "Given the plurality of often conflicting values that can be brought to any discussion of priorities in health care, it is positively undesirable (as well as foolish) to search for some set of principles that will make our decisions for us."[4] So does David Hunter: "Rationing will always be a messy affair. We should not seek to deny the mess but accept it."[5]

Thus, since "ought implies can" and explicit rationing seems practically impossible, we are said to be stuck with implicit rationing.

The argument from the utility of ignorance

The second argument against explicit healthcare rationing derives from health economics[6] and emphasises the emotional consequences of explicit rationing. Explicitly to confront individuals with the fact that, because of scarce resources, they will not receive health care that they need will make them more unhappy than believing that there is no clinical option but to take what is offered. This distress will be compounded if they discover that other patients deemed more worthy of resources will receive treatments denied them.[7] Two noted health economists have described the "deprivation utility" of being kept in ignorance in such circumstances.[8]

This idea can be extended to healthcare rationers themselves. Telling patients they will not receive appropriate clinical care for economic reasons is stressful, more so than pretending that the treatment will be futile or just not mentioning it at all.[9] As a result, it is again argued, on utilitarian grounds, that implicit rationing makes more sense than that which is explicit.

The argument from bureaucratic and political effectiveness

A third defence focuses on the bureaucratic and political difficulties that are said to accompany explicit rationing. Attempting to strike the right balance between competing claims for funding within health authorities is not easy, and the same argument holds for central government attempting to weigh up conflicting demands on the public purse. In such circumstances complaints by the public about the management of explicit rationing will certainly make life more difficult for those responsible for organising health care. Much better then to continue the myth that decisions about the allocation of such care are based on clinical criteria alone.

Hunter, for example, has supported such mythology: "The public is more likely to accept rationing decisions made by doctors rather than managers and politicians."[5] Clinical discretion in rationing is essential given the diversity of individual cases. If the public becomes aware that more general value judgments—say about cost effectiveness, moral desert, and quality of life—are behind rationing decisions then such discretion may be undermined. Letting the cat out of the bag would then advantage articulate patients who will know how to play the now transparent system. "Lack of visibility", Klein argues on the same note, "may be a necessary condition for the political paternalism required to overcome both consumer and producer lobbies".[10]

Similar arguments have been developed by Mechanic, who worries that explicit rationing might jeopardise the stability of the political process surrounding health care. He speaks of the "many disaffected people" created by the knowledge of why resource decisions are being made about them and others; whose responses would not be "conducive to stable social relations and a lower level of conflict; and who are likely to confront government and the political process with unrelenting agitation for budget increases".[11] Much better for people to believe—even if it is false—that rationing decisions are inevitable for purely clinical reasons. Then clinicians, managers, and politicians can get on with the job of making decisions in what they believe to be are the best interests of patients. Explicit rationing "will inevitably result in acrimony difficult to manage politically".[11]

Clear criteria for explicit rationing do exist

It is hard to believe that anyone really thinks that we should not at least try to understand the criteria that should be used in rationing decisions—to make them explicit in this sense and to compare them with criteria actually used. Refusing to make this attempt is tantamount to giving up the possibility of evaluating either the justice or the efficiency of the rationing process, of accepting that healthcare resources should be distributed in ways which might do as much harm as good.

Against the background of the explicit moral foundations of the NHS, such pessimism is curious. For in general terms, nothing could be clearer than the ethical principles at the heart of the health service. The most well known and important of these principles is that there should be equal access to health care within the NHS based on equal need.[12] The first group of critics might be claiming that there is something inherently confused about the equal need–equal access equation. Conversely, they could be claiming that, even if the formulation is clear in principle, in practice it is so bereft of organisational and procedural content that it is of little use to those who must work in the real world of managerial, economic, and moral expediency. Both of these claims are false.

As regards the first claim, suppose that we define the need for health care as the requirement for specific clinical intervention in order to avoid or to minimise sustained and serious disability.[13] What would it mean to suggest that we have no clear understanding of what this means in practice? It is what occurs in the delivery of health care at its best on a daily basis throughout the world. To be sure, there are disagreements about the appropriateness or efficacy of some interventions, diagnoses, and prognoses.[2] But this does not detract from the clarity of what we do know or the success of the service that is often delivered. Those who like to emphasise the uncertainty of medicine will no doubt change their tune when they contract serious and treatable illnesses.

There is similar clarity associated with moral arguments for providing access to appropriate health care on the basis of need. Our potential to flourish as individuals in whatever cultural environment depends on our ability either to participate within or to struggle against it. We require the help of others if we are to discover what we are capable of doing and becoming. Sustained and serious disability inhibits our capacity to interact with and learn from others and is thus in the interests of everyone to avoid if possible.[13]

But this is just another way of underlining how vital it is for those so disabled that appropriate health care be distributed on the basis of need and on no other individual attribute.[14] On a macro level this means that healthcare resources should be allocated to local populations on the basis of the most accurate needs assessments of which we are capable. This means that generally speaking, resources should be divided proportionally between the different types of disabling and treatable illnesses represented within such populations. Specific types of illness should not be discriminated against on the grounds of popularity or estimations of social worth. Rationing should take place within rather than between different areas of healthcare need.[15]

On the one hand, disabling disease may strike any of us without warning and if health care is distributed on any other basis, most of us cannot know for sure whether or not we may individually qualify for it. On the other hand, it is in our interests that those known and unknown persons on whom we socially depend for our potential to flourish will also be kept as healthy as possible. Rationally, therefore, we should want for others what we desire for ourselves.[15]

The concepts of equality of need and of access to health care based on it are also reasonably straightforward. Once it is accepted that the focus of any definition of healthcare need should be associated disability and that

142

the macro allocation of resources should take place accordingly, the issue of equality on the level of micro allocation partly reduces to what levels of disability can coherently be deemed to carry with them the same moral entitlement to health care. It also partly concerns how we can ensure that those who are believed to be in such equal need can be assured an equal chance of benefiting from whatever clinical resources are available for its satisfaction.

Triage is the procedural embodiment of the belief that some levels of disability caused by illness are morally similar enough to warrant the same priority of access.[16] When triage is linked to a system of waiting which ideally gives each person within each category of urgency an equal chance of treatment—one based on a first come first served basis—then equal access to available resources will be seen in principle to be provided on the basis of what is accepted to be equal need.[15] A trip to any well run accident and emergency department will provide ample practical illustration.

Of course, people may accept such principles in theory yet argue that in practice they become so muddled as to reduce to confusion. Such arguments confuse substantive and procedural moral issues.[17] Moral principles must be interpreted to apply them to specific problems, and unless there are procedures to optimise the rationality of such interpretation, confusion and injustice can indeed follow. For example, the assessment of healthcare need is often based on questionable methods, including ad hoc extrapolations from prior levels of clinical demand.[18] Further, the traditional organisation of surgical waiting lists tells us more about the clinical preferences of surgeons and strategies for queue jumping than the just distribution of treatment to patients.[19]

Thus confused organisational practices do not necessarily entail confusion within the moral principles which are supposed to inform them. They can also reveal the inability or unwillingness of rationers to take clear principles seriously, or to recognise the rights of patients in whose interests they are supposed to be acting. We should direct our energies to correcting this problem rather than wringing our hands about the inevitability of methodological and administrative chaos.

Of course, further effort is required to show how theory and practice can be better integrated, and the clarity of theory will benefit as a result. This is the aim of current attempts to create uniform guidelines for clinical diagnosis and treatment, and similar research should be undertaken on various aspects of rationing—for example, triage and fair waiting patterns for different conditions, the non–provision of life saving treatment, the determination of clinical futility.[20] Those who support implicit rationing rightly argue that it will be a difficult task.[2] However, theoretical clarification and consistent practice will continue to elude us unless decision makers

143

are encouraged to make explicit and publicly defend the criteria for rationing which they do use.

The disutility of ignorance: micro rationing should be explicit

The second argument made against explicit rationing embraces the utilitarianism of traditional health economics. Thus it suffers from the same blindness to issues of equity as other attempts to reduce rationing decisions to the aggregate calculation of preference—for example, QALYS (quality adjusted life years).[15] The key argument is the same: explicit micro rationing will ultimately create more unhappiness—less utility—on the part of both patients and doctors than implicit rationing.

There is nothing new about the idea that, because patients may find certain types of information distressing, they should not be told it. Yet any benefit derived from deception will be sustained only while patients are kept in ignorance. If they discover that they have been deceived, their sense of betrayal will probably far outweigh any distress from being told the truth.[21] Therefore, it can just as convincingly be argued that utilitarian clinicians should pretend that they take seriously the right of patients to be told the truth, even if in reality they do not. Indeed, evidence suggests that this is precisely what patients wish, including those who are terminally ill.[22]

Similar arguments apply to the suggestion that patients will be less distressed if they are not told about the real reasons why they are denied treatments. Such a discovery could again lead to considerable unhappiness when the deceit is discovered; we cannot calculate the utilitarian outcome of deceit with any certainty. Of course, if we take seriously the right of patients to protest against rationing decisions then such deception will be unjustifiable in any case.

That clinicians will be happier if they keep patients in the dark about the realities of rationing is just as questionable. This argument works only if it is assumed that the deception will always be successful. Yet, because we cannot be sure of the outcome, sustaining deception over time can itself be distressing, especially if patients begin to ask more direct questions about why they are not receiving care which they have heard is available to others. Also, because their professional guidelines so consistently emphasise the duty to respect the autonomy of patients, good clinicians are increasingly taught to feel uneasy about any form of deception not invited by patients in advance. In any case, to base a decision on the well being of the clinician rather than the best interests of the patient would be unacceptable.

144

Macro rationing should be explicit

Within a democracy an informed public can undoubtedly give administrators and politicians a hard time. Yet citizens should have explicit information about any policies which can dramatically affect their lives.

First, as John Stuart Mill saw so clearly, unless citizens are given at least the potential for such influence, their own moral development will be damaged: they will not have the same personal stake in either learning about or conforming to the rules of their culture. More specifically, their moral commitment to democracy itself will be undermined. If we accept that democratic participation in public and political life is a good worth pursuing then it follows that the citizenry should be educated about the matters on which their participation is sought.[23]

Second, informed democratic feedback can improve the effectiveness of public policies through allowing policy makers more accurately to assess the results of their labour. It also helps to make them more reflective, knowing that they may be held to account by those whose interests they are supposed to serve. Such accountability is particularly important in the light of the tendency for vested interests to dominate the formation and implementation of policy.[13]

More informed public understanding and participation should aid rather than impede the efficiency, accuracy, and equity of healthcare rationing through enabling more accurate needs assessments, more effective audit, and more representative research.[24] This will help to ensure that macro policy aims are being achieved and that the moral boundaries of acceptable rationing are not being exceeded in the name of expediency. Reasonable levels of understanding and participation will also help to minimise distress in the face of non–treatment. This is because the degree of scarcity and the reasons for it will be explicit, along with the knowledge of how and when resources are being distributed between different areas of clinical demand.

The fact that the public has been oblivious to healthcare rationing in the past may well explain some traditional allegiance to the NHS. Such ignorance undoubtedly made the work of health care much easier than it would otherwise have been. Yet it also has led to injustices—for example, ageism and arbitrariness in the construction and management of waiting lists.[19,25] That cat is now out of the bag, and the media will see that it is not put back. The argument for implicit macro rationing on the grounds of bureaucratic and political stability is just unrealistic.

The same argument is also paternalistic, illegitimately conflating a professed concern with the public welfare with bureaucracies' love of secrecy. The key premise is that the public will not be able to understand and therefore not be able to accept the degree of indeterminacy and

145

inaccuracy which necessarily accompanies decision making about healthcare rationing.

As regards health care, there seems little convincing evidence that this is so. When anger and frustration do occur, it is usually in the face of the harm caused by what is perceived to be a mistake falling outside the boundaries of what is regarded as acceptable error. Citizens in the UK have traditionally drawn such boundaries generously. Mistakes and inaccuracy in themselves have usually been tolerated, provided that they are publicly acknowledged and that serious attempts are made to detect why the problems arose and how they will be avoided in future.[26]

Conclusion

I have argued that none of the arguments against explicitness in healthcare rationing is convincing. Attempts to clarify the moral principles on which rationing should be based are not doomed to failure. We already know what these principles are: we must now have the moral courage to develop them further to ensure that they form the explicit basis for rationing decisions at both micro and macro levels. There is too much secrecy in British public life already. It should be reduced rather than sustained within the NHS.

1 Maxwell R, ed. *Rationing health care.* London: Churchill Livingstone, 1995.
2 Klein R, Day P, Redmayne S. *Managing scarcity.* Buckingham: Open University Press, 1996; 83–93, 102–8.
3 House of Commons Health Committee. *Priority setting in the NHS: purchasing.* London: HMSO, 1995:57.
4 Klein R. Dimensions of rationing: who should do what? *BMJ* 1993;**307**:309–11.
5 Hunter D. Rationing health care: the political perspective. In: Maxwell R, ed. *Rationing health care.* London: Churchill Livingstone, 1995:877–84.
6 Coast J. Rationing within the NHS should be explicit: the case against. *BMJ* 1997;**314**: 1118–22, 148.
7 Hoffenberg R. Rationing in action. *BMJ* 1993;**306**:198–200.
8 Mooney G, Lange M. Ante-natal screening: what constitutes benefit? *Soc Sci Med* 1993; **37**:873–8.
9 Fuchs V. The "rationing" of medical care. *N Engl J Med* 1984;**311**:1572–3.
10 Klein R. Dilemmas and decisions. *Health Manag Q* 1992;**14**:2–5.
11 Mechanic D. Dilemmas in rationing health care services: the case for implicit rationing. *BMJ* 1995;**310**:1655–9.
12 Davey B, Popay, J. *Dilemmas in health care.* Buckingham: Open University Press, 1993: 27–42.
13 Doyal L, Gough I. *A theory of human need.* London: Macmillan, 1991:49–75;297–312.
14 New B, LeGrand J. *Rationing in the NHS.* London: King's Fund, 1996:63.
15 Doyal L. Needs, rights and equity: moral quality in health care rationing. *Qual Health Care* 1995;**4**:273–83.
16 Winslow G. *Triage and justice.* Berkeley: University of California Press, 1982.
17 Doyal L. Medical ethics and moral indeterminacy. *J Law Soc* 1990;**17**:1–16.
18 Curtis S, Taket A. *Health and societies.* London: Arnold, 1995:138–80.
19 Frankel S, West R. What is to be done? In: Frankel S, West R, eds. *Rationing and rationality in the National Health Service.* London: Macmillan, 1993:115–31.

20 Grimshaw J, Hutchinson, A. Clinical practice guidelines—do they enhance value for money in health care? In: Maxwell R, ed. *Rationing health care*. London: Churchill Livingstone, 1995.
21 Beauchamp T, Childress J. *Principles of biomedical ethics*. New York: Oxford University Press, 1994:395–406.
22 Davis H, Fallowfield L. *Counselling and communication in health care*. London: Wiley, 1991: 3–24.
23 Gutman A. *Liberal equality*. New York: Cambridge University Press, 1980:48–63.
24 Pfeffer N, Coote A. *Is quality good for you?* London: Institute for Public Policy Research, 1991:45–58.
25 Grimley Evans J. Health care rationing and elderly people. In: Tunbridge M, ed. *Rationing health care in medicine*. London: Royal College of Physicians, 1993.
26 Audit Commission. *What seems to be the matter: communication between hospitals and patients*. London: HMSO, 1993:1–75.

A rejoinder to Len Doyal

JOANNA COAST

Doyal's paper takes three arguments for implicit rationing in health care and attempts to refute each, while simultaneously advocating explicitness on two main grounds. Doyal's first reason for advocating explicit rationing is that it allows the pursuit of particular rationing criteria, specifically the criterion of equal access for equal need. His second reason is that explicit rationing allows individuals to maintain their moral commitment to democracy and participate in healthcare rationing, leading to increased justice. Doyal further refutes the notion that disutility may be associated with explicit rationing on the grounds that any deceit of the public could lead to even greater disutility as this deceit becomes known and the public feels a sense of betrayal. This brief critique looks first at the intrinsic contradiction between Doyal's two main grounds for explicitness before considering each in isolation. Doyal's arguments relating to the potential for disutility resulting from explicit rationing, which address the major part of my paper, are then discussed.

In reading Doyal's paper, it is difficult at times to separate the general argument for explicitness in rationing from the argument for a *particular system* of explicit rationing. Perhaps this is inevitable. Explicitness may not itself be a virtue except insofar as it improves the basis upon which healthcare rationing is carried out, with such improvement inevitably being dependent upon the particular scheme adopted. Unfortunately, however, Doyal's two arguments are to a large extent contradictory. On the one hand, he is quite certain about the appropriate principle for rationing health

147

care—equal access for equal need; on the other, he advocates explicitness as a means of pursuing democratic participation among the citizenry. Yet does not democratic participation imply that a quite different, and possibly (to Doyal) morally unacceptable, scheme of rationing could result?

Doyal does not accept any impossibility in defining workable criteria for rationing. In fact he advocates the specific criterion of rationing on the basis of equal access for equal need. Although Doyal professes the simplicity of this criterion, both in theory and in practice, he glosses over a number of issues. He begins by advocating the allocation of healthcare resources at a macro level on the basis of needs assessment, with resources being divided proportionately between the different types of disabling and treatable illnesses (on what basis is unclear: numbers of individuals affected? severity of disability? resources required to treat a particular number of individuals?, etc). Interestingly, however, it appears that Doyal does not consider this to be rationing, stating "Rationing should take place within rather than between different areas of healthcare need"—perhaps he is arguing in favour of implicit rationing at this level! At the micro level Doyal states that the issue of explicitness reduces to defining the levels of disability that can be deemed to carry with them the same moral entitlement to health care. This would seem to be a major undertaking.

Doyal's arguments for explicit rationing on the basis of increased moral commitment are based on a particular ideology. They contain a number of unsubstantiated claims for explicitness, for example, the assertion that "reasonable levels of understanding and participation will ... help to minimise distress in the face of non–treatment". Doyal also links implicitness to injustice, stating that ageism has resulted from the obliviousness of the public to healthcare rationing. Yet democratic participation of the public in rationing could easily result in increased ageism (and hence injustice) rather than a reduction.

Doyal relies heavily on the notion of deceit: that implicit rationing involves actively deceiving the public and that the disutility associated with explicit rationing arises entirely from abandoning ignorance/increased knowledge. Doyal argues that choosing not to ration explicitly at every level means that the public could ultimately experience greater disutility (resulting from a sense of betrayal) upon finding out about rationing than they would with an initial state of explicit rationing. However, although ignorance may be a sufficient condition for increased utility via implicit rationing, it may not be necessary. There is the further possibility that equivocation among the public is enough to maintain the utility associated with not having explicit rationing. Turning a blind eye to healthcare rationing may be preferable to its full acknowledgment, given the disutility that may result from explicitness.

My argument is that we should not wholeheartedly embrace explicit rationing without first finding out more about the potential harm that could result. A system of explicit rationing could cause individuals disutility and ultimately produce more costs than benefits. Given his moral commitment to democratic participation, it is perhaps surprising that Doyal is not a greater advocate for finding out whether the citizenry would prefer implicit or explicit rationing.

The case against

JOANNA COAST

This paper must begin with some definitions. Implicit rationing of health care occurs when care is limited and where neither decisions about which forms of care are provided nor the bases for those decisions are clearly expressed.[1] Hence it is the unacknowledged limitation of care. Explicit rationing is, unsurprisingly, the opposite: decisions about the provision of health care are clear, as are the reasons for those decisions. Nevertheless, the term explicit has been used in various ways, from Klein's version of explicit rationing as rationing by exclusion,[2] to a more general concern with honesty and openness surrounding the context of healthcare rationing.[3]

Both types of rationing decision can be made at different levels. Various taxonomies have been used, but this paper will assume four distinct levels of priority setting: across whole services; within services but across treatments; within treatments; and between individual patients.[1] It is at the last level, particularly, that explicit rationing may be most troublesome.

Currently, rationing in the UK at all levels is predominantly implicit.[4,5] It is carried out by doctors who are aware of the resources available and who ration by telling patients that they cannot help them, rather than explicitly stating that resources are not available.[4,6-9] The denial of care is instead made to seem optimal or routine.[4,10] Hence there is little sense among the public that healthcare rationing takes place on a daily basis. Indeed, on those occasions when explicit rationing is perceived (particularly at the level of the individual patient)—for example, in the case of child B[11,12]—there tends to be public outcry about the introduction of rationing.

The proposition put forward, that rationing should be made explicit at all levels of NHS decision making is very much "today's topic". An impetus in favour of explicit rationing has built up among both academics and healthcare policy makers. The assumption seems to be that explicit rationing is a wholly good thing—implying openness and honesty, and consequently

149

paving the way to a more equitable, efficient, fairer service in which the public can also democratically influence the process and outcome of rationing.

There are, however, problems with this view, which tend to fall into one of two categories. First, the assumption is that the path towards explicit rationing is one that it is practical and possible to follow. Many commentators have, however, questioned this, arguing that implicit rationing may be preferable to imperfect explicit rationing.[2-14] Second, there are some levels of healthcare decision making at which it may be intrinsically undesirable to make rationing explicit. This is because explicitness in rationing may cause various members of society to experience disutility. I will concentrate mainly on the second of these two broad areas of difficulty although I will first cover briefly the arguments relating to the practicality of explicit rationing.

Is explicit rationing practical?

The challenges to explicit rationing on the grounds of practicality fall into two broad areas. One relates to the possibility of developing explicit rationing schemes, the second to the practicalities associated with implementing and sustaining such schemes.

Advocates of explicitness are particularly concerned that the principles on which rationing is based should be established, yet it may not be possible to obtain consensus about such principles. Klein and colleagues suggest there is no obvious set of ethical principles or methodologies on which to base rationing, given the large number of objectives that healthcare is required to pursue simultaneously.[2,15] Indeed, "it is positively undesirable (as well as foolish) to search for some set of principles or techniques that will make our decisions for us".[2]

Further, it may be impossible to sustain explicit rationing given the potential impact on the stability of the healthcare system.[10] Individual strength of preference for health care is not accounted for by explicit rules, and disaffected individuals with a strong preference are unlikely to accept easily explicit rationing not in their favour.[10] This argument is associated with Mechanic, who states that such challenges will weaken the resolve of health authorities to continue with explicit rationing of health care and will, instead, force them to return to more flexible, implicit means of rationing care. The work of Redmayne et al,[15] which shows that UK purchasing authorities who attempted to rule out certain procedures have since relaxed such exclusions, is used to illustrate this problem.[13] Hunter, too, points out that, by increasing the visibility of the decision process, the potential for conflict among decision makers is likely to increase, resulting ultimately in a conservative approach in which current patterns of provision would be preserved.[14]

Disutility associated with explicit rationing

Utility is an economist's term, representing the idea of preference for a particular state—for example, we are likely to have a higher preference for a treatment that leaves us mobile and pain free than for one that leaves us walking with a stick and in severe pain. Economists would say that the first treatment provides higher utility than the second. Disutility is merely the opposite of utility.

Economists traditionally associate utility only with the purchase of goods and services. Similarly most economists working in the area of health care have conventionally associated utility only with the outcome of treatment and not with the process by which either the treatment or the healthcare service is provided. The concern here is that there may be aspects of disutility associated with the process of explicit rationing that are not associated with implicit rationing.

Let us first clarify some of the important aspects that might characterise explicit rationing. The citizenry as a whole would be aware that the rationing is taking place. They would essentially be either colluding with some form of technical rationing scheme—for example, based on combining information about cost with that about treatment outcome—or be directly involved in rationing through some form of public consultation process. Whichever the alternative, the citizenry would inevitably feel some of the responsibility for the denial of particular forms of treatment. Ultimately this means denial of treatment to particular individuals. (With openness and public debate, inevitably responsibility follows: if the citizenry knows about rationing and the principles on which it is based then it has the choice over whether to collude with these principles or to oppose them. With any rationing scheme some individuals will be denied care: the choice of individual will depend on the particular rationing scheme.)

In order to have explicitness at the doctor–patient level, general practitioners would be obliged to explain to patients not being referred for treatment that the reason for lack of referral is lack of resources, and for some reason (lower need, lower effectiveness, high cost, reduced "deservingness", age) they are the patients who will not receive treatment. Similarly, hospital doctors would have to explain to emergency patients (and their friends and relatives) that resources are not available for treatment and (as above) that this particular patient is the one who will not receive treatment. In some cases patients will subsequently die. Given the emergency nature of some illnesses, appeals may not be possible because of time constraints.

151

Explicit rationing may therefore give rise to two particular sources of disutility. First, citizens becoming involved in the process of denying care to particular groups of individuals or particular individuals may experience disutility (denial disutility). Second, disutility may result when particular individuals are informed explicitly that their care is being rationed (deprivation disutility). The important question here is whether such disutility could potentially outweigh any increases in utility associated with beneficial changes in who is treated which might result from explicit rationing.

Disutility associated with denial

Denying treatment to patients who are sick and who may die or live years with disability might be expected to cause a considerable amount of disutility to those having to make this decision. Under implicit rationing, the doctor will make the decision about which of two individuals should receive treatment. Aaron and Schwarz, in their examination of implicit rationing in the UK, show that doctors deal with resource limits by seeking medical justification for their decisions.[4] In fact: "Doctors gradually redefine standards of care so that they can escape the constant recognition that financial limits compel them to do less than their best."[4]

Currently the disutility that results from denying patients is experienced primarily by doctors but is minimised by the doctor's ability to justify, both personally and to the patient, the absence of treatment on medical grounds. The decision can then be conveyed to the patient by a variety of means. Options for treatment can just not be mentioned, or they can be stated to be inappropriate for particular reasons. If patients are not referred, they will not be rejected from care, and the doctor will not then have to face the rejected patient.[4]

Contrast this with explicit rationing. Whatever the form of explicit rationing, the citizenry are now aware that they have some responsibility for denying treatment to some individuals and there is some evidence that such treatment may cause the citizenry disutility. As Callahan states: "This anguish will be all the greater when the victims are visible and when the accountability for their condition cannot be evaded."[16]

Those conducting explicit priority setting exercises have often found a general reluctance to specify services to be denied. For example, attempts at programme budgeting and marginal analysis have shown that, although happy to decide what should go on an incremental wish list, groups are much more unwilling to identify services for explicit disinvestment.[17–19] Similarly, reluctance to deny services was noted during initial consultation on core services in New Zealand.[20] Instead: "There is considerably more support for alternative approaches to expenditure constraint. ... High

152

technology treatments and pharmaceuticals expenditure are usually cited as examples."[20]

Although increases in denial disutility felt by the citizenry could be expected to be offset by reductions in disutility on the part of the doctor, this is unlikely to be the case. With explicit rationing doctors would still be responsible for informing patients that they were unable to receive treatment, and would be unable to justify this denial on medical grounds. The disutility associated with denying the patient could actually be much greater for the doctor: "For physicians to have to face these trade-offs explicitly every day is to assign to them an unreasonable and undesirable burden."[21]

Disutility associated with deprivation

Rationing of health care, whether implicit or explicit, inevitably means that some individuals will receive treatment and some individuals will not. Let us imagine two patients, A and B, who could each receive equally beneficial treatment. Rationing, however, means that only one patient can receive treatment within the resources available.

First assume the current system of implicit rationing. Patient A is treated and patient B is not. Patient B is told that there is nothing that can be done for her. A receives an improvement in health, and therefore an increase in utility, and B's utility does not change. Neither A nor B is aware that a rationing decision is being made: they do not have perfect knowledge about the availability of medical technologies and are unaware of the possibilities for treatment. B may feel pleased that A has received care and is left with hope that treatment for her condition might be developed.

Now assume an explicit rationing system. Patient A again receives treatment at patient B's expense, but now this fact is known to both individuals. As before, A receives utility from treatment and B's utility related to treatment does not change. Is there a difference between implicit and explicit rationing? Conventionally the answer to this question would be no: the outcome is the same in both scenarios. But B now knows that a treatment exists that is not being provided to her. She is likely to feel resentful, as well as being aware that there is no hope. It is quite believable that B will experience a feeling of deprivation and hence disutility.

This notion of deprivation disutility was first developed by Mooney and Lange in relation to antenatal screening.[22] They discuss deprivation disutility in terms of women ineligible for a screening programme who subsequently bear a child with the disability for which screening was available. These women may well experience a loss in utility compared with women bearing a healthy child, but this loss in utility may be greater because they know that the screening test could have informed them about the disability, allowing them to choose how to proceed at an earlier stage.

The essence of deprivation disutility is that it derives from knowing that something could have been done, but was not. As Evans and Wolfson point out: "It is easier to bear inevitable disease or death than to learn that remedy is possible but one's personal resources, private insurance coverage or public programme will not support it."[23]

The notion of explicitly informing patients that their care is being rationed has been considered inhumane. For example, Hoffenberg has stated that where doctors have to treat some patients with a particular illness at the expense of others he would prefer to see implicit rationing, "not through a belief in medical imperialism or paternalism but through a concern about the anguish that patients and their relatives might feel if they knew that they are being denied services that other patients had received explicitly because of cost".[24]

In practice, the fact that patients are seldom informed that they will not receive treatment because resources are not available provides the main indication for the existence of deprivation disutility. (The main exception to this is where elective patients are told that if they wish to receive treatment of a particular type then they must pay for it, the most obvious example being in vitro fertilisation for infertile couples.) Instead, denial of treatment is made to seem routine or optimal, for example (italics added): "By not referring the patient, the doctor spares the *nephrologist* from having to say no *and the patient and family a painful rejection.*"[4]

Deprivation disutility resulting from implicit rationing may extend beyond the patient directly involved, to the population more generally. Individuals may feel deprivation disutility not only for themselves but also altruistically on behalf of others, particularly close friends and family. When care is explicitly rationed, particularly potentially life saving care for young children, donors often provide the required funding for the treatment to go ahead—for example, a single donor paid for the required treatment in the Child B case.[12] This is the case even when charitable donations made more generally could be expected to provide much greater benefit to society as a whole and hence would appear to be more efficient. Deprivation disutility felt on behalf of others could explain such donations.

Discussion

Arguments for explicitness in healthcare rationing, as with the arguments against, are many and varied. Some are ideological and relate to the intrinsic benefits of honesty and openness—for example, the development of individuals' moral commitment to democracy and the discouragement of vested interests.[25] Others are more closely linked to the notion that explicitness will lead to an improvement in decision making[25] and ultimately a healthcare system that provides a greater total benefit to society. Economists, particularly, have placed a strong emphasis on explicit rationing techniques which aim to maximise the benefit available from healthcare resources.

Those advocating explicit rationing would generally expect an improvement in decision making to result, at least indirectly, from such explicitness. This is essentially equivalent to saying that the utility to society as a whole would be increased as a result of explicit rationing. There is no evidence, however, that this would be the case. For practical reasons, the benefits of explicitness may be less than expected. Explicitness may be unable to generate the sets of principles that lead to improved decision making. Even if such principles can be generated, it may not be possible to sustain the explicit decisions that follow. Further, the advocates of explicit rationing have ignored the potential for disutility arising from this very explicitness. Such disutility may affect both those making the decisions to ration care and those being denied. In particular, explicitness at the level of the individual patient is likely to lead to substantial disutility, which may itself outweigh any potential benefits in terms of improved outcomes or improved equality.

Greater total utility may therefore result from the equivocation associated with implicit rationing than from the openness and honesty of explicitness. It is questionable whether decisions about rationing should be made explicit at all levels of NHS decision making (unless this position is held on purely ideological grounds). In fact, whether rationing should be explicit (particularly at the level of the individual doctor–patient consultation) is an empirical question, the answer to which must ideally be determined on the basis of considering the various utilities associated with implicit and explicit rationing. It is important to determine the extent of increased utility which could, in practice, be expected to result from explicitness (via improved decision making). Furthermore, it is important to estimate whether such increased utility would be substantially offset by the disutility associated with deprivation and denial, the magnitude of which may be significant and has still to be determined. Researchers and health authorities should be exploring these issues rather than jumping on the fashionable bandwagon of explicit rationing.

1 Coast J, Donovan JL, Frankel SJ, eds. *Priority setting: the health care debate.* Chichester: Wiley, 1996.
2 Klein R. Dimensions of rationing: who should do what? *BMJ* 1993;**307**:309–11.
3 New B, Le Grand J. *Rationing in the NHS. Principles and pragmatism.* London: King's Fund, 1996.
4 Aaron HJ, Schwartz WB. *The painful prescription. Rationing hospital care.* Washington, DC: Brookings Institution, 1984.
5 Grimes DS. Rationing health care. *Lancet* 1987;**i**:615–6.
6 Dean M. Is your treatment economic, effective, efficient? *Lancet* 1991;**337**:480–1.

7 Klein R. Rationing health care. *BMJ* 1984;**289**:143–4.
8 Parsons V. Rationing: at the cutting edge. *BMJ* 1991;**303**:1553.
9 Smith R. Rationing: the search for sunlight. *BMJ* 1991;**303**:1561–2.
10 Baker R. The inevitability of health care rationing: a case study of rationing in the British National Health Service. In: Strosberg MA, Weiner JM, Baker R, Fein IA, eds. *Rationing America's medical care: the Oregon plan and beyond.* Washington DC: Brookings Institution, 1992:208–29.
11 Price D. Lessons for health care rationing from the case of child B. *BMJ* 1996;**312**:167–9.
12 Toynbee P. Did the NHS cheat Jaymee? *Independent* 1995;27:Oct. 23.
13 Mechanic D. Dilemmas in rationing health care services: the case for implicit rationing. *BMJ* 1995;**310**:1655–9.
14 Hunter D. *Rationing dilemmas in healthcare.* Birmingham: NAHAT, 1993.
15 Redmayne S, Klein R, Day P. *Sharing out resources. Purchasing and priority setting in the NHS.* Birmingham: NAHAT, 1993.
16 Callahan D. Ethics and priority setting in Oregon. *Health Affairs* 1991;Summer:78–87.
17 Cohen D. Marginal analysis in practice: an alternative to needs assessment for contracting healthcare. *BMJ* 1994;**309**:781–4.
18 Donaldson C. Commentary: possible road to efficiency in the health service. *BMJ* 1994;**309**:784–5.
19 Donaldson C, Farrar S. Needs assessment: developing an economic approach. *Health Policy* 1993;**25**:95–108.
20 The Bridgeport Group. *The core debate. Stage one: how we define the core. Review of submissions.* Wellington: Department of Health, 1992.
21 Fuchs VR. The "rationing" of medical care. *N Engl J Med* 1984;**311**:1572–3.
22 Mooney G, Lange M Ante–natal screening: what constitutes benefit? *Soc Sci Med* 1993;**37**:873–8.
23 Evans RG, Wolfson AD. *Faith, hope and charity: health care in the utility function.* Vancouver: University of British Columbia, 1980.
24 Smith R, ed. *Rationing in action.* London: BMJ Publishing Group, 1993.
25 New B, on behalf of the Rationing Agenda Group. The rationing agenda in the NHS. *BMJ* 1996;**312**:1593–601.

A rejoinder to Joanna Coast

LEN DOYAL

Joanna Coast has written a robust defence of implicit rationing, by which she appears to mean the intentional deception of patients and the public about the real reasons why they have been denied scarce resources. She argues that being explicit about rationing may make patients and clinicians feel bad and interfere with the plans of policy makers. Coast outlines reasons for believing that the aggregate "disutility" derived from keeping patients and the public in the dark outweighs whatever utility might be gained from rationing in ways that are more explicit, honest, and transparent.

My paper offers two types of reasons why Coast's arguments should be rejected. First, utilitarian justifications of implicit rationing can just as easily be employed to justify rationing that is explicit. Second, public deception in the name of increased utility is immoral in any case. It violates the moral right of citizens to information relevant to the determination of their individual and collective destinies. Let us take each argument in turn.

It is now widely accepted within medicine that deception can create more disutility than telling the truth—for both patients and clinicians. For example, patients may well be *more* distressed to discover that they have not been told the truth about their condition, prognosis, or treatment than they would have been had they not been kept in ignorance. By and large, the evidence suggests that patients want such information. Nothing Coast argues makes me think the situation is different with respect to healthcare rationing.

In her defence of implicit rationing, Coast does offer one piece of hard evidence to the contrary. Some studies have shown that citizens are unhappy about participating in the denial of specific types of care to other citizens. This is taken to imply that they would rather such denial occur implicitly and without their knowledge. However, such evidence can just as easily be interpreted as showing that citizens are unhappy at participating in explicit rationing that is perceived to be unfair. Explicit rationing that is perceived to be equitable—along the lines, say, outlined in my paper—may well evoke a more favourable response. Certainly, patients waiting in accident and emergency departments appear quite content to make judgments about preventing access to patients who they believe are trying to jump the queue!

So even on utilitarian grounds, I think that the evidence—such as it is—pulls against Coast's arguments for implicit rationing. This is not, however, the *main* reason why I favour explicit rationing.

Second, I state in my paper, "if we take seriously the right of patients (or the public) to protest against rationing decisions then (implicit rationing) will be unjustifiable in any case". It follows from Coast's arguments that the right to such informed protest, along with the right to informed participation in the political process, can justifiably be ignored as regards health care, provided that the result is to increase the marginal balance of happiness over unhappiness.

Aldous Huxley saw in *Brave New World* the nightmare of a society organised along these lines—a world where major priority is indeed placed on minimising the stress of the population and exercising social control to this end. Here, human autonomy and dignity are sacrificed on the altar of a conception of human interests which does not incorporate either. In my view—and I am sure that of many others—the avoidance of such a nightmare is well worth the toleration of a great deal of "disutility". Morally, any that might be associated with explicit rationing is well worth the price.

11 Direct public and patient involvement in rationing

The following three contributions are not framed in a 'for and against' format. The authors felt that the topic—essentially concerned with democratic participation—was not suited to oppositional debate. Instead, Anna Coote and Heather Goodare stress the possibilities for increasing public and patient involvement, while Len Doyal warns that there are moral boundaries to these apparently uncontroversial propositions.

Possibilities for direct public involvement in rationing decisions

ANNA COOTE

Should the views of the public be directly taken into account in making rationing decisions? I shall argue that there are strong grounds for doing so. But first a number of points must be clarified. What do we mean by "rationing decisions", who are "the public" and what is meant by "directly taken into account"?

My argument concerns rationing decisions within the NHS. I shall not labour the point that rationing decisions are necessary. The amount of public money available to pay for public health services is and will continue to be limited. Even if more money were voted to the NHS by taxpayers, there would always be more that could be done to augment and improve health services. Decisions would still have to be made about how to spread the money around. Rationing in this context means the fair distribution of resources, not just "cuts".

By "the public" I mean ordinary members of the community who may or may not have experience as patients of the NHS. These are the people for whom the NHS is intended: people who have a right to vote when they are 18 and a duty to pay taxes when they are employed—you, me, our families, friends, and neighbours.

What is meant by taking the views of the public "directly into account"? I take this to mean that the views of the public are canvassed explicitly and

158

considered seriously. They carry weight in the process of decision making. This does not mean that they dictate the outcome of rationing decisions. It is not *direct* democracy that is called for, but *participative* as well as *representative* democracy.

I shall argue, first, that it is appropriate that the views of the public be taken into account. Next, I shall argue that it is necessary for the public to be more directly involved than at present. I shall then indicate how it is possible to do so effectively.

Why is it *appropriate* for the views of the public to be taken into account?

There are two main reasons: first, the NHS must be rendered genuinely accountable to the public and, second, rationing decisions are essentially political in nature.

As a publicly funded organisation, providing services for the public, in the public interest, the NHS is widely acknowledged to owe accountability to the public. But how is that achieved? John Stewart[1] has argued persuasively that accountability is not guaranteed merely by democratic election; it is a two way process. He distinguishes between *being held to account* and *giving an account*.

Both are necessary for the full expression of accountability. Being held to account is enforced through the election process and is necessarily periodic. Accounting is equally important to the continuing relationship of stewardship and should involve not just the giving of an account but listening to what is said.

Accordingly, the accountability of a public authority requires a continuing exchange or dialogue with the electorate in which the public can both obtain and provide information, while the authority is open to scrutiny, listens, and responds. This process informs the authority's decision making between elections as well as voters' choices at election time. In this way, active, participative democracy may be seen as complementing and validating representative democracy.

But should all health service business be subject to a continuing dialogue with the public? Broadly speaking, there are three main categories of decision that are made within the health service. Those that are mainly clinical in nature draw upon the particular expertise of doctors and nurses. Executive decisions require managerial and administrative skills, including legal and accounting skills, which must often be combined with clinical expertise. Decisions concerning the values and goals that shape and drive the NHS require not only clinical and executive know-how but also—and essentially—political understanding. This category of decision is about defining the public interest in the NHS: what the service stands for in the eyes of the public and what it is expected to achieve for the public.

The NHS is accountable to the public for the outcome of all its decisions, but only in the third category can the "full expression" of accountability be appropriate. The public at large cannot intervene in clinical or managerial matters, because ordinary people lack the necessary expertise and because the system would be unworkable if every detail were subject to public debate. But when it comes to decisions about the meaning and purpose of the NHS, the views of the public must be taken into account. In a democracy, the people have a right to make political decisions.

Rationing decisions fall into this category because they concern the fair distribution of resources. Deciding what is "fair" requires a political understanding about the meaning and purpose of the NHS. If, for example, the NHS had been set up explicitly to deal with accidents and emergencies, there would be no need to allocate NHS funds to primary health care or to preventive medicine. If it were intended to serve only those covered by health insurance policies, there would be no need to decide how the NHS should cater for the uninsured. But as the service is intended to be universal and free at the point of use, aiming to promote better health for all, as well as to treat illness and injury, these objectives must help to determine what is a "fair" allocation of resources, and what is not.

There is nothing new about rationing in the NHS. It is simply being done more openly than in the past and by different people, so that the political nature of decisions has become more apparent. Since the birth of the NHS, doctors have had to decide whether it is worth treating this patient or that, or giving this treatment or that. Costs as well as clinical possibilities influenced their decisions. But the process was covert and the distinction between professional and political judgment was fudged. When the 1991 NHS reforms shifted some of the burden of decision making to managers, that helped to bring decisions about rationing out into the open. NHS managers, unlike doctors, cannot hide behind the doctrine of clinical autonomy. But from where can they derive legitimacy for their decisions? Lawyers and auditors will decide whether they are operating with probity, but the law does not specify how resources are to be rationed, so managers must seek the approval of those who have a democratic right to decide what is "fair".

Why is it *necessary* for the public to be more involved than at present?

There are two main reasons why greater public involvement is necessary. First, current arrangements are inadequate, leaving the public without effective channels of communication. Second, public confidence in the

NHS is eroding and the best hope of restoring it lies in building an open and mature relationship between ordinary citizens and decision makers. The actual connection between the public and policy making on health is tenuous.[2] Most decisions are taken, within a framework set by government, at local levels, by individual health authorities, GP fundholders, and provider trusts. Choices are made and implemented every day of the year. In so far as they are accountable for their decisions, the authorities, GPs, and trusts must answer to the Secretary of State for Health, who in turn answers to Parliament. Every 4–5 years, the public can vote for a new Parliament and, possibly, for a new government. This is the only direct power that the people currently have to shape decisions about health. Less directly, they elect local authorities, many of which have health committees. Two further mechanisms (non-executive directors of health authorities and trusts, and Community Health Councils) provide severely limited opportunities for indirect public participation. Beyond that, there is only the power of protest or persuasion: by lobbying or demonstrating, by attending public meetings, and by responding to opinion surveys people can say what they think. Whether the decision makers listen, hear, or take heed is up to them. The weakness of current mechanisms for public accountability becomes increasingly problematic as the political salience of rationing decisions intensifies. I shall not dwell here on the question of whether or not the NHS faces a "doomsday scenario", with shrinking resources unable to meet escalating demands. The important point is that more and more people think there is a problem. The media have become increasingly interested in the state of the NHS. A steady flow of stories about declining standards, regional variations, and individuals who are treated inappropriately or refused treatment have helped to fuel public concern.

More generally, a growing sense of injustice and insecurity has eroded public confidence in the NHS. Public attitudes have displayed increasing scepticism about the efficacy of the state and politicians' ability to keep their promises. A similar sense of uncertainty has extended to science and medicine, tempering faith in their infallibility. More people are aware that governments, despite their claims to the contrary, are unable to protect them from major risks (to their health and environments, in particular) associated with technological change. More people are having to accept that doctors do not always know what is best for them, because of the limitations of medical science. Some are beginning to suspect that doctors will not always do what is best for them because they are influenced more by commercial than by clinical values.

The more uncertain and suspicious people become about the capacity of politicians and "experts" to protect them against risks, the more likely they are to be fearful for the future. People are less certain that paying taxes and national insurance for a working lifetime will guarantee them the health care they need when they need it. One consequence is that those who can afford it are, increasingly, tempted to exit from the NHS for non-emergency treatment and "go private". They buy the right to jump queues, to get treatments that might otherwise be denied them, or for which they would have to wait. This not only creates a two tier service with better services for the better off. It breaks the bonds of common interest and mutuality that bind people together. It begins to destroy that sense of a shared investment in services that all citizens own and need. This is the route to social fragmentation and conflict, to a thinning and fraying of the fabric of democracy—a development that can already be seen in the USA.

The life and soul of the NHS depend on public trust. Trust is increasingly acknowledged as a key component in management, and most especially in large organisations that are intended to serve the public interest. It is important in the NHS because the activity of production in medical care is so often identical to the product. Some critics have argued that an organisational culture based on trust reinforces the authority of doctors and the primacy of the "medical model" of health care. But this is missing the point—our aim should not be to resuscitate the power relations of the unreformed NHS, but to forge a new configuration of trust based relationships to serve the goals of a twenty-first century health service.[3]

Trust can no longer be built on a paternalistic system in which "doctor knows best", which claims to protect and provide, but fails to consult or involve the public in decisions. It requires mutual understanding and respect, rather than dependency or any imbalance of power. In a high trust organisation, the underlying assumption is that *all* those involved share common aims and are, broadly speaking, willing and competent to play their part in achieving them. This implies a mature, adult-to-adult relationship between patients and doctors, as well as between citizens and those who plan and shape the service.

Is it *possible* to take the views of the public directly into account in rationing decisions—and to do so effectively?

Resistance to the notion of public involvement in rationing decisions often stems from uncertainty about how this can be achieved and to what effect. It is widely assumed by those who routinely take decisions that ordinary members of public lack the capacity to grasp complex issues or to form views of any relevance, that they are too gullible and will believe anything they read in the popular press, that their views are inevitably shaped by narrow and selfish concerns, and that they are generally apathetic and will not take the time or trouble to consider anything that does not affect them directly and personally. In short, they are stupid, untrustworthy,

162

and irresponsible, and it is too hazardous to attempt to take their views into account.

Much turns on *how* the public's views are canvassed, and *on what aspects* of rationing decisions. I do not suggest that the public should be directly involved in decisions about individual cases. These should be left to the clinicians. However, the clinicians' decisions about individual patients should be made within a common framework of criteria and procedures, aimed at ensuring the fair distribution of resources.[4] This framework should be established at a national level to promote fairness and consistency across the country, but should be sufficiently flexible to allow for local interpretation, taking account of local needs and conditions. The views of the public should be taken into account in determining both the national framework and local priorities, because these require not only technical skills but political understanding.

Various methods may be applied in order to canvass public views. Among the most commonly used are opinion polls and public meetings. Focus groups and health panels have been introduced more recently by some health authorities. Citizens' juries were piloted by health authorities for the first time in 1996. Taking just these four examples, each has its strengths and weaknesses. Opinion polls can reach substantial numbers of people relatively cheaply and can be scientifically verified if the sample is large enough. But they are superficial and reflect the *uninformed* views of the public. Public meetings are open and offer the chance for an exchange of views, but they are often poorly attended and then only by those individuals who have a particular interest in some aspect of the agenda. Focus groups are a useful source of qualitative research data, and can help to probe public opinion in more depth than opinion polls, but they provide little opportunity for informed deliberation, and they remain a tool in the hands of the researchers, who are free to interpret the findings to suit their own ends. Health panels can involve larger numbers over a sustained period, giving the panel members a chance to become more informed about their subject but, like focus groups, they are open to manipulation and, in addition, there is a danger of panel members developing too cosy a relationship with the health authority that convenes it.

Citizens' juries represent an attempt to overcome some of these difficulties.[5] They provide an opportunity for a representative sample of between 12 and 16 members of the general public to spend four days considering a policy question, scrutinising information, cross examining witnesses and discussing the matter among themselves. There is a world of difference between views forged in this context and views expressed through polling data, which can only convey a snapshot of popular opinion. According to the model developed in the UK pilot series, the jury is independent of the commissioning authority and owns the report which sets out its conclusions. The jury's decision is not binding, but the health authority is expected to respond within a set time and either to abide by the jury's recommendations or to explain publicly why not. Experience to date[5] suggests that in these conditions jurors are able to understand complex and technical subjects, and to adopt a responsible, community perspective, becoming confident and competent decision makers on behalf of their fellow citizens. On the down side, juries are open to accusations of bias unless recruitment and moderation techniques are scrupulously open and fair. They are an elaborate and relatively expensive form of public involvement, costing up to £16 000 each. The process aims to combine *information, time, scrutiny, deliberation, independence* and *authority*. Most other forms of opinion research and public involvement have some of these features. What is distinctive about citizens' juries is the package: the model is designed to ensure that all features are present to a substantial degree. It provides for a *democratic dialogue* between members of the public and those who make decisions in the public interest.

It is important to identify and to try to create conditions that are conducive to open, informed, and interactive decision making. We may seek to achieve these either through the particular model of the citizens' jury, or through others currently being tested or yet to be invented or refined in future. My point is not that the citizens' jury is the best or only way of enabling the public to form and articulate views, but that effective public participation in rationing decisions is not only appropriate and necessary, but also demonstrably possible.

1 Stewart J. *Innovation in democratic practice.* Birmingham: Institute of Local Government Studies, 1995.
2 Cooper L, Coote A, Davis A, Jackson C. *Voices off: tackling the democratic deficit in health.* London: IPPR, 1995.
3 Coote A, Hunter D. *New agenda for health.* London: IPPR, 1996.
4 Lenaghan J. *Rationing and rights in health care.* London: IPPR, 1996.
5 Coote A, Lenaghan J. *Citizens' juries: theory into practice.* London: IPPR, 1997.

Possibilities for direct patient involvement in rationing decisions

HEATHER GOODARE

Why should patients be directly involved in decisions about their care? And in helping to decide priorities? I shall argue that the patient is ultimately

164

the most important person in the decision making process. Whose body is it anyway? And perhaps, even more importantly, whose mind? In the words of Anne Dennison (an ovarian cancer patient): "What I want from my doctor more than anything else is the recognition that I have a mind."[1] I shall focus particularly on the field of cancer, which is where my personal experience lies.

In no other area, I believe, are patients allowed so little autonomy in decision making. This, it seems, results more from the problems that health professionals have in talking about cancer than from genuine difficulties in facing reality on the part of patients. In some countries people are still not even told that they have cancer. But it is a common disease: in the Western World one in three of us will have cancer at some point in our lives, and one in four will die of it. Why is the incidence of cancer on the increase? Where should we really concentrate our efforts—on treatment or on prevention? Does our Western greed with its disastrous impact on the environment lead to degenerative diseases that could easily be prevented? These are the questions asked by the patients I meet. Many of them ask for more resources to be put into public health measures that will help the next generation and protect their daughters and sons: clean water, clean air, less use of pesticides, more respect for the plant and animal kingdom, less prescription of drugs, particularly hormones, for humans and animals alike, better health education, and better housing. Ivan Illich argued as long ago as 1976: "the cost of therapy for cancer caused by exhaust fumes could be added to each gallon of fuel, to be spent for cancer detection and surgery or for cancer prevention through anti-pollution devices . . .".[2]

When it comes to treatment rather than prevention, again the solutions asked for are simple, and would be cost effective if patients were listened to. Involve the patient in healthcare decisions and you may actually save money. "A service responsive to the needs and wishes of patients is one where patients are fully involved in their health and health care. Knowledge about health, illness, symptoms and treatment gives people more control over their circumstances, and helps them access and use services effectively".[3] For such a patient centred service to be developed, the following are necessary.

Doctors should listen to patients

There is a consensus among all political parties that the NHS should be primary care led.[4] This puts a heavy responsibility on general practitioners. Diagnosis is difficult, but people know their own bodies, and persistent symptoms should not be ignored. I have heard too many stories of breast lumps dismissed with the comment "Oh my dear, you're far too young to have breast cancer". Yet the disease can be found in women as young as

165

20.[5] Late referral to a specialist results in more expensive treatments and earlier death.[6,7] Also, patients are now becoming more litigious, and refusal to refer resulting in serious consequences will only be more costly in the long run for the NHS that ultimately picks up the bill. We are not talking here about the "jam" (procedures such as breast augmentation or tattoo removal), but the bread and butter: urgent treatment for what may turn out to be life threatening disease.

Doctors should be honest with patients

When it comes to treatment for cancer, patients are rarely given the evidence for the effectiveness of the treatments they are asked to undergo, or information about their side effects. But patients do want this information.[8]

It seems that the main problem preventing doctors from sharing information with their patients is their reluctance to be completely honest about prognosis. This would mean acknowledging and communicating some of the uncertainty and the pain of knowing that the patient may die quite soon and that treatment may only prolong the agony.

Here we are faced with a genuine dilemma. It appears from some studies that patients will go for very toxic treatments that have only a very slim chance of success.[9] Hope springs eternal! But a recent study shows that the problem may in fact be one of communication. For those with malignant cerebral glioma "Severely disabled patients gain little physical benefit from radiotherapy, whereas those not so disabled may experience considerable adverse effects."[10] This was the doctors' view.

But when the patients were interviewed:

> Most patients with malignant glioma initially seemed unaware or only partly aware of the poor prognosis. Relatives were more aware, more distressed, and often concerned to protect patients from full awareness, which made it difficult to explore with patients directly the possible trade off between quality and length of life. Conceptualising the question as a rational choice ignores the social and emotional context of life threatening disease.[11]

It is clear from this paper that the reason 43% of patients did not know their poor prognosis was that the surgeons had not told them.

Denial is a useful defence mechanism for cancer patients, and can sometimes be helpful (as Steven Greer and colleagues showed in their study of coping styles and breast cancer).[12] But denial in doctors is more serious if it leads to a situation where patients, relatives, and clinicians are involved in a costly *danse macabre* where people weave in and out of each other and nobody is telling the truth. As Illich points out, it is a delusion that "ongoing rituals that are costly must be useful".[2]

I have found in my work as a counsellor that couples experience profound relief when they are finally able to communicate with each other, acknowledge the reality of the situation, and share their fears, plans for the future (whatever it may be), and love for each other. The close of a long life together is not the time for dissembling. They may decide to go for further treatment, but if the clinician has been honest with them and they know that this is palliative rather than curative, then the emotional energy expended on pretence can be diverted into more constructive channels—making the best of the time that is left, seeing to unfinished business, and so on. In some cases they will decide to refuse further orthodox treatment but go for some kind of complementary care, which may at least make them feel better. Many would argue that such treatments, which are very cheap compared with radiotherapy or chemotherapy, should be available on the NHS. Many such therapies are offered by hospices: aromatherapy, counselling, massage, acupuncture for pain relief, and so on.

Maher observes that treatment, erroneously seen as "curative" by patients, is often used as a substitute for communication, and that there is a failure to refer early enough to palliative care teams.[13] So in the area of treatments for advanced cancer, money might well be saved if the evidence for efficacy (or lack of it) were actually acknowledged and shared with the patients. This strategy could be seen as "rationing", but in my view it would be a more rational use of resources, and one that patients and their relatives would endorse and appreciate.

In another field, that of treatment for depression, there is plenty of evidence that many patients prefer counselling or other forms of talking therapy to drug treatments, and that they may well be more effective, and cost effective, in the long term.[14-17] Another cheap and apparently effective alternative to drug therapy is exercise on prescription, now being tried out in many centres, modelled on the Hailsham experiment in West Sussex.

Patients should share responsibility with clinicians

The right to participate in decision making also involves responsibility. If clinicians are prepared to share power they can be relieved of some of the responsibility for outcome. This may require a culture change, but one that a mature, democratic society should welcome. Patients might, for example, take responsibility for keeping their own medical records (as recommended recently in a report commissioned by the Chief Medical Officer for Scotland): this could improve the efficiency of out-of-hours doctors' visits.

Having more information not only helps people have a greater say in the way health care is provided, it also helps them make more appropriate and responsible use of services and take greater responsibility for their own health.[3]

Also, crucially, "Better informed patients will not necessarily demand more resources".[3] For example, too many routine checkups for cancer patients waste time and money,[18][19] but if these are to be reduced in number, patients need more information about possible symptoms to watch out for, and easy access to a streamlined service should they need it.

Increasingly, patient opinion is being sought in policy making. The stated ambition of the British NHS is to aim for "a high-quality, integrated health service which is organised and run around the health needs of individual patients, rather than the convenience of the system or institution".[3] A service designed around the needs of individuals is less wasteful of resources. For example, patient preferences for home births and home deaths wherever possible should be respected—and money for high-tech hospital facilities thereby saved.

An example of patient influence on purchasing decisions is the 1996 *Guidance for purchasers: improving outcomes in breast cancer.* Partly as a result of patient input, important items were included in the recommendations: particularly the provision of psychosocial support, which is still patchy. Early psychosocial intervention prevents long term morbidity and thus saves money. Another example of rationalisation recommended in the *Guidance for purchasers* is the prescription of tamoxifen, which tends to be done wholesale, regardless of oestrogen receptor status, which is rarely assessed. It is wasteful to prescribe tamoxifen for someone who is unlikely to benefit, and at least one group of patients has now been identified in this category: women under 50 whose tumours are oestrogen receptor negative.[20] Such women would only experience the side effects, some of them life threatening, for no benefit. It makes good economic sense to spend a small amount on the hormone assay (which is done routinely in countries such as the USA, although not yet in Britain), and save on prescription of the drug and further treatments to alleviate its side effects. But, in the UK, most patients still have to ask for this simple test—if indeed they know it exists. Basic information is still needed to enable patients to know which questions to ask, and they should not have to fight to get this information.

Here again this is an area where patients, not clinicians, are the experts. It is clear that patients given information about possible side effects do not go on to imagine them,[21] yet eminent clinicians still argue that side effects are "overstated" or "anecdotal".[22]

A recent prospective study found that patients experienced the side effects of tamoxifen as "worrying", and that the degree of distress occasioned by such symptoms was differently evaluated by health professionals and

168

patients, with oncologists in particular liable to underestimate the distress to patients.[23]

Another important treatment area is radiotherapy, which certainly has its place, particularly in palliative care. But it is widely used as adjuvant therapy in early breast cancer, and patients are hardly ever given full information about the long term risks and late effects, although the facts are well known to clinicians. Patients are not happy to discover that their bodies secretly harbour an iatrogenic time bomb.

A surgeon wrote in 1991:

> Our knowledge as to which patients to treat is poor, but we do know that overall survival is unaffected by radiation given early to all, rather than later to those who need it . . .[24]

In 1995 a meta-analysis confirmed that adjuvant radiotherapy for breast cancer conferred no long term survival advantage.[25] But patients are not told this, and so huge sums of money continue to be spent on treatment, and women expend their own energy, time, and resources on attending for radiotherapy, with its associated morbidity (early and late), forgoing productive work and costing the state unnecessary benefits. Given appropriate information, many patients are perfectly competent to make their own decisions about treatment. Some may prefer to accept radiotherapy on the grounds that it may help to prevent local recurrence (deliberately choosing the short term view), but some may well decide to keep it in reserve in case a problem occurs later. They may also have a view on the short term inconvenience of daily low dose treatment with low morbidity versus less frequent attendance for high dose treatment with greater risk of long term complications, requiring expensive salvage therapy.[20]

Conclusion

So, involving patients in decision making does not necessarily imply increased expenditure: it may actually involve less. The same goes for designing clinical trials: Bradburn and colleagues have shown that asking patient opinion at the design stage of trials can iron out difficulties, improve recruitment, and save both time and money.[27]

These principles of partnership with the patient could be applied to all forms of health care in fields other than cancer, and decision making should be equally shared, taking into account all the evidence. If "rationing" is an issue, then this should be stated clearly, so that the individual patient can "shop around" if she or he wishes. If the general practitioner does not offer counselling, say, or osteopathy, the patient may prefer to find a doctor who does. I have argued that the individual patient's view should be taken into

169

account in making rationing decisions. The first step is to give the patient honest information. Traditionally, British people have accepted with gratitude and without question what the NHS has to offer. Now that market forces have come into play, patients are beginning to demand value for what is, after all, their own money collected through taxation. She (or he) who pays the piper should call the tune.

Further than this, the autonomy of the patient should be respected in a more radical way. With the erosion of paternalism that goes with genuine democracy, "people will limit medical therapies because they want to conserve their opportunity and power to heal. They will recognise that only the disciplined limitation of power can provide equitably shared satisfaction".[2] The equitable sharing of both satisfaction and resources is surely what we all desire—patients, clinicians, and managers. But in the global context, where, for instance, a cataract operation in India or Africa may cost as little as £12 (US$18), petty squabbles about who is going to pay for expensive and often ineffective interventions seem appallingly trivial. The healthcare rationing debate needs to be widened to the world itself if we are to deserve our place on the planet for generations to come.

1 Dennison A. What do I want from my cancer doctor? In: Slevin M, Short R, eds. *Cancer and the mind. Br J Hosp Med conference supplement.* London: Mark Allen, 1990.
2 Illich I. *Limits to medicine. Medical nemesis: the expropriation of health.* London: Marion Boyars, 1976; Penguin Books, 1990.
3 Department of Health. *The National Health Service: A service with ambitions.* London: HMSO, 1996 (Cm 3425).
4 Cole M. A united stance on the future of health. *Hosp Doctor* 1996; 14 November.
5 Dale E. The lump. In: Duncker P, Wilson V, eds. *Cancer: through the eyes of ten women.* London: HarperCollins, 1996.
6 Burgess CC, Ramirez AJ, Richards MA. Who and what influences delayed diagnosis of breast cancer? *Proceedings of the British Psychosocial Oncology Group.* London: December 1993.
7 Martin IG, Young S, Sue-Ling H, Johnston D. Delays in the diagnosis of oesophagogastric cancer: a consecutive case series. *BMJ* 1997;314:467–71.
8 Fallowfield L, Ford S, Lewis S. No news is not good news: information preferences of patients with cancer. *Psycho-oncology* 1995;4:197–202.
9 Slevin ML, Stubbs L, Plant HJ, Wilson P, Gregory WM, Armes PJ et al. Attitudes to chemotherapy: comparing views of patients with cancer with those of doctors, nurses, and general public. *BMJ* 1990;300:1458–60.
10 Davies E, Clarke C, Hopkins A. Malignant cerebral glioma—I: Survival, disability, and morbidity after radiotherapy. *BMJ* 1996;313:1507–12.
11 Davies E, Clarke C, Hopkins A. Malignant cerebral glioma—II: Perspectives of patients and relatives on the value of radiotherapy. *BMJ* 1996;313:1512–16.
12 Pettingale KW, Morris T, Greer S, Haybittle JL. Mental attitudes to cancer: an additional prognostic factor. *Lancet* 1985;i:750.
13 Maher EJ. Giving hope to patients with advanced disease. *Cancer care: more than medicine,* Conference, Brighton, 11–12 October 1996. London: British Association of Cancer United Patients, 1996.
14 Priest RG, Vize C, Roberts A, Roberts M, Tylee A. Lay people's attitudes to treatment of depression: results of opinion poll for Defeat Depression Campaign just before its launch. *BMJ* 1996;313:858–9.
15 Scott AIF, Freeman CPL. Edinburgh primary care depression study: treatment outcome, patient satisfaction, and cost after 16 weeks. *BMJ* 1992;304:883–7.

16 Mynors-Wallis LM, Gath DH, Lloyd-Thomas AR, Tomlinson D. Randomised controlled trial comparing problem solving treatment with amitriptyline and placebo for major depression in primary care. *BMJ* 1995;**310**:441–5.
17 Parish A. Depressed? I was just totally fed up. *Hosp Doctor* 1996; 14 November.
18 Gulliford T, Opomu M, Wilson E, Hanham I, Epstein R. Popularity of less frequent follow up for breast cancer in randomised study: initial findings from the hotline study. *BMJ* 1997;**314**:171–7.
19 Radford JA, Eardley A, Woodman C, Crowther D. Follow up policy after treatment for Hodgkin's disease: too many clinic visits and routine tests? A review of hospital records. *BMJ* 1997;**314**:343–6.
20 Cancer Guidance sub-group of the Clinical Outcomes Group. *Guidance for purchasers: improving outcomes in breast cancer*. The Manual. NHS Executive (96 CC 00 21), 1996.
21 Lamb GC, Green SS, Heron J. Can physicians warn patients of potential side-effects without fear of causing those side-effects? *Arch Intern Med* 1994;**154**:2753–6.
22 Baum M, Cuzick J. Adjuvant treatment with tamoxifen [letter]. *BMJ* 1996;**312**:1036.
23 Leonard RCF, Lee L, Harrison ME. Impact of side-effects associated with endocrine treatments for advanced breast cancer: clinicians' and patients' perceptions. *The Breast* 1996;**5**:259–64.
24 Clark A. A surgeon's experience of breast cancer. In: Clark A, Fallowfield L, eds. *Breast cancer*. London: Routledge, 1991:11.
25 Early Breast Cancer Trialists' Collaborative Group. Effects of radiotherapy and surgery in early breast cancer: an overview of the randomized trials. *N Engl J Med* 1995;**333**: 1444–55.
26 Bradburn J, Maher J, Adewuyi-Dalton R, Grunfeld E, Lancaster T, Mant D. Developing clinical trial protocols: the use of patient focus groups. *Psycho-oncology* 1995;**4**:107–12.

The moral boundaries of public and patient involvement

LEN DOYAL

The NHS does not have enough resources to meet the healthcare needs of all British citizens. Therefore, rationing within the health service is inevitable.[1] We live in a democracy where citizens should be able to participate in decision making about issues that affect their vital interests. We therefore need to ask what role the public should have in determining who gets what. The government has endorsed the importance of public participation in setting priorities in health care spending, as have other commentators.[2–4] In this chapter, I will argue that although the involvement of the public is crucial for the effective and efficient practice of health care in this country, it has a limited role in decision making about healthcare

171

rationing. Some forms of rationing will be shown to be morally wrong, irrespective of their actual or potential popularity.

The importance of democratic participation in public life

Democratic forms of social organisation presuppose two things: that citizens have a right to participate in the way in which they are governed and that they all have this right in equal measure. Historically, the primary moral justification for equal rights was protection from the arbitrariness of despotism. Yet this concern was balanced by anxiety about extending citizenship to the poor and uneducated who might exercise their democratic rights irresponsibly. The extension of suffrage in Europe was accompanied by a growing recognition that it was unreasonable to expect people without political experience to support democracy unless they were given the right to learn and mature through participating in it.[5]

Current writers on democratic participation in the formulation of public policy make the same point.[6] Despite the existence of universal suffrage, the creation and implementation of such policy increasingly occurs in the face of public passivity. This is hardly surprising. Many citizens feel that all they can do to exercise their democratic rights is to elect politicians who then become outside their democratic influence. Elections themselves can cover so many issues that local concerns about specific issues become lost in the generalities of party politics.[7]

Methods have been proposed to deal with this problem through involving the public more in local decision making. They include citizens' juries, issues forums, and deliberative opinion polls on national issues, as well as other approaches to create consensus and shared vision among groups seeking a voice in local policy formation. All of these approaches recognise that citizen led democracy must be informed to be effective.[8] Citizens' juries, for example, involve the selection of representative individuals from different social groupings to whom resources are made available for educated and reasoned debate on particular issues. Jurors have a more direct stake in policy formation than ordinary voters because their conclusions must receive a formal and public response from the authorities that organise them.[9]

Such innovations in the theory and practice of democracy are to be applauded. Decisions about public policy have been dominated for too long by experts with specialised knowledge of types of human need, but little awareness of how these are experienced by individuals in varying circumstances. This top down control engenders political passivity as well as stifling the bottom up feedback required for monitoring the effectiveness, efficiency, and fairness of policy decisions. A dual strategy of democratic

172

representation is required which includes both expert and experiential understanding in policy formation.[10]

Yet it does not follow from the importance of expanding democratic participation in the political process that local majorities should be given unlimited scope about what they decide on behalf of others. To be fair, few have explicitly argued for such an approach. However, justifications for constraining the power of local democracies have usually focused on their inadequate resources for proper deliberation (for example, poor access to all relevant information). The implication is that the power of the public should be greatly increased were these problems to be resolved.[11] Here I wish to argue in principle for limits to be set on such power. However effective local democracy may be in eliciting informed participation, there will still be boundaries of democratic decision making which should not be crossed unless democracy itself is to be undermined. To see why, we must consider the role of the public in rationing health care within the NHS.

Public participation in healthcare rationing: the problem

There can be little doubt that the NHS faces serious problems of scarcity—of not having enough resources to meet growing demand.[12 13] Many health authorities have had to make swingeing cuts over the past year, and some trusts are close to bankruptcy. Bed numbers and clinical sessions have been reduced to the point that in many areas no elective interventions are being performed. Although patients with serious conditions are being kept waiting for unacceptable, and sometimes for agonising, periods of time, ways are also being found to keep patients in need off waiting lists altogether. The problems accumulate.

Some commentators continue to argue that such indicators do not necessarily represent a crisis in NHS funding. However, the fact remains that Britain continues to spend less per capita on health care than other comparable developed nations.[14] There is little doubt that many citizens in obvious need of health care have had to do without—either altogether or for long and distressing periods. Many who receive care from the NHS and most who work in it agree that resources are scarce and times are hard.

Of course, there is nothing new in all this: the health service has never had enough to go around.[15] What is new is the volume of apparently unmet need and the increasingly public character of the rationing that now occurs. Before the most recent Government reforms, rationing decisions were often camouflaged as clinical judgments rather than what they generally are—judgments by clinicians that may or may not be morally acceptable.

Through the internal market they now become the responsibility either of purchasers charged with meeting local need through designated budgets or of clinicians responsible for allocating patients to assigned clinical sessions.[15] For the first, the Government has dictated that the criteria employed for macro allocation should be transparent and that the public should have a voice in their determination.[2] Micro allocation between individuals continues to remain clouded by the myth of moral neutrality in the exercise of clinical judgment.[16]

A variety of democratic initiatives has occurred in healthcare planning which mirrors the more general approaches to local democracy already described. Attempts have been made to organise groups of citizens to solicit their views about (among other things) how much spending should be directed to different areas of clinical care. This has included debate about whether some areas should receive no funding at all and be excluded from the NHS tariff.[17 18] These initiatives as well as opinion polls on the same topic have yielded similar lists of clinical conditions deemed either not worthy of medical treatment or much less worthy than other conditions.[19 20] Equally, local groups have debated whether or not the risky lifestyle of some individuals should qualify their right of equal access to health care.[17]

It has become clear that such public consultation can be biased by the way in which policy questions are selected and worded for consideration, by who presents the options to be considered and, of course, by the socioeconomic background of the participants themselves.[21] Yet the underlying message of some commentators and health authorities remains the same: provided that these problems can be tidied up, representatives of the public should be able to participate in decisions about which areas of health care are funded and who should receive that care. Is this an acceptable position?

Good citizenship and the equal right to health care

We have seen that arguments supporting public participation in the formation of social policy link it to the exercise of good citizenship. It is through such participation that citizens improve their potential contribution to democratic decision making. Yet some social policies are not compatible with good citizenship because they place arbitrary limits on the personal capabilities required to be a good citizen.[22] Even the majority should not be allowed democratically to ration health care if the result is artificial constraints on the ability of the minority to be good citizens.

Whatever our cultural environment, we evolve and flourish as individuals through our social interaction with others—through our potential for successful social participation. It is through interaction with others that we learn and have reinforced those cognitive and emotional skills that constitute

174

our personal identity. The more we can and do engage in social participation, the more we learn about who we are and what we are capable of. This in turn will enable us to optimise our contribution to the very social processes from which we have derived personal benefit. Thus, anything that disables the potential for successful social participation counts as fundamental harm to those individuals involved.[10]

Such disability is frequently the result of serious physical and mental illnesses which prevent individuals from engaging in successful social participation. Such illness renders individuals less able to act and interact in ways that characterised their private and public life before illness. Their ability to join, continue, or improve their democratic participation in the political process will also be compromised. Illness not only harms the sick individual but also the democratic polity that cannot benefit from their potential contribution. Thus it is self defeating in the name of more effective democracy to allow one group of citizens to restrict the access of others to needed health care.[10]

The fact that such a group may constitute a majority of decision makers is irrelevant if its decisions about rationing undermine the ability of members of the minority to be the best citizens they can. And the irrationality does not stop here. To allow majorities to dictate the health care received by minorities is imprudent for all citizens. Aside from the very wealthy, we all live under a veil of ignorance as regards the financial impact of unforeseen serious illness. Members of majorities may think that they will never contract disabling illness which they identify with the unlikely misfortune of minorities. Fate may dictate otherwise. As so many Americans have recently learned, individuals can never be sure of fair access to needed health care without (1) universal cover and (2) the certainty that no one can arbitrarily strip them of it.[23]

Allowing the public to jeopardise the physical and mental security of their fellow citizens is not only irrational; it is dangerous. If most citizens are allowed to deny unpopular treatments to members of minorities in serious need—or to individuals whose lifestyles do not find favour—where will it end? If the only justification is that this is what the majority prefer, then it would follow that it would be just as appropriate for the majority to deny treatment to the sickest 1% of the population. And if 1%, why not 10%? If the comeback is that the British would never engage in such injustice, the fact is that they already have. Some treatments are unavailable on the NHS tariff in one sixth of health authorities.[24]

Paradoxically, the rejection of the right of a majority of the public to restrict resources to a minority will make the need for rationing more acute—even as regards that minority. In such circumstances, the fairness of the distribution that does occur becomes of the utmost importance. It was against the background of arguments concerning citizenship of the sort already outlined that fairness within the NHS became defined by one

175

substantive moral principle: equal access to scarce resources on the basis of equal need.[25] The procedural implications of this principle (which I have discussed at length elsewhere) are that scarce resources should be allocated as follows.[26]

To meet need in proportion to its distribution within the population—This distribution should be documented through needs assessment that is properly resourced and as accurate as possible. Epidemiologically, need should always be linked to evidence of serious disability in relation to social participation and better ways should be found to measure this.

Without prejudice to the type of need or the health care appropriate to its satisfaction—Rationing should occur within and not between components of health care. Social participation can be seriously impaired by any one of a range of conditions for which treatment has not found public favour (for example, certain types of infertility). Those with these conditions have the same moral claim on resources as anyone else.

According to moral similarity based on extremity of need—Such similarity is determined through improved methods of triage which should always be linked to assessing levels of impaired social participation. Those in most serious need should be treated first. Criteria other than urgency and similarity of need should be rejected.

So that there is equality of access based on extremity of need—The implementation of such access should occur through the administration of fair waiting lists among those with morally similar needs. This method of distribution is fair because it is a form of randomisation based on the time of appearance and seriousness of need—the "lottery of nature"—rather than other personal attributes.

Only for treatments of potential effectiveness—Medical or surgical intervention may be futile because of the untreatable condition of specific patients or general lack of clinical success. Offering such treatment in the face of either circumstance is inequitable because it wastes resources that could potentially be employed in the successful care of others.

Without reference to the lifestyle of recipients—Choices of lifestyle are shaped by different levels of understanding, emotional confidence, and social opportunity which are determined by varying social backgrounds that are partly beyond the control of the individuals concerned.

A real commitment to an optimally successful democracy based on equal rights of participation demands support for the fair delivery of optimally successful health care to all citizens within that democracy. This commitment should be no more subject to alteration by the public than by the purchasers and providers who currently run the health service.[27]

Finally, substantive moral and procedural principles on their own solve few problems and principles for rationing health care are no exception. They must be interpreted, and there will be disagreement about how to implement them in practice—for example, about where to draw the line between minor and serious disability and between different categories of triage. For the moral goals of the health service to remain intact, such disagreements must be resolved as rationally as possible. Rules of representation, communication, and debate are required which ensure relevant knowledge of the problem at hand, minimise the influence of arbitrary vested interests, and maximise the opportunity for all participants to express their views.[10] If the goal is an optimally rational and moral health service, these further procedural rules of communication also designate the boundaries beyond which democratic decision making should not be allowed to proceed.

The positive role of public participation in health care

The arguments advanced above against allowing democratic majorities to determine the substance or procedure of healthcare rationing do not entail that the public has no role in healthcare planning and monitoring. Their participation and experiential understanding are crucial.[26] Examples of this include the following.

Better needs assessment—We require much more accurate epidemiological information about the scope and types of serious disability faced by local populations.[28] Also required is more conceptual and empirical clarification about the ways in which such disability is operationalised, especially in relation to its impact on the potential for successful social participation. Without the involvement of patients, carers, relatives, and friends, this will be impossible.[29]

Better audit and research—The clinical satisfaction of the basic need for physical and mental health will always occur against the background of current understanding of best treatment. It is now clear that the evidence base for such understanding is often lacking and that audit and research are vital components in both the efficient and effective use of resources. Neither form of investigation is possible without the active participation of the public. Indeed, they have a particularly important role for the public in suggesting new enquiries which might not otherwise be apparent to

177

health professionals too close to their immediate clinical and research interests.[30]

Better defence of patients' rights—Patients are concerned about more than the clinical effectiveness of treatments on offer. They also expect that their autonomy will be taken seriously, particularly their right to informed consent and confidentiality. The participation of the public—through triggering the various avenues of complaint and regulation and active involvement in subsequent enquiries—is crucial for moral audit of this aspect of clinical practice to be effective.[31]

More equity—Where consistency with first moral principles does not prevail, inequity will result. This may be because the experiences of the recipients of health care are not sufficiently reflected in policy decisions about resource allocation. When inequity does occur, the public has a crucial role to play in highlighting its existence and in making political demands through appropriate democratic channels that it be stopped. There is no doubt that such channels need to be improved and that the criteria employed for rationing should be made explicit and open to public scrutiny.

The moral foundations of the NHS are not up for democratic grabs and its principles must be applied consistently to individual cases. In the process, rules of rational communication and debate must be respected and not altered as the result of public opinion or political pressure. Within this framework, the goal of an equitable health service can be achieved with the active participation and support of the public.

Consequences for the participation of individual patients in rationing decisions about themselves

We have argued that the public should not be the final arbiter of decisions about rationing health care. Similar arguments hold in the case of individual patients making demands on scarce resources. Estimates of the severity of disability associated with specific illnesses will be impossible without effective communication which accurately elicits and records the experiences of patients. Equally, patients' perceptions of the success of clinical interventions in reducing disability will be of importance for their own future prognosis and treatment, as well as adding to the evidence base of such intervention for others. The success of such communication will partly depend on the trust and the spirit of partnership that develops (or fails to do so) between patients and their clinical advisers.[32]

However, it does not follow from the importance of communication for a good clinical relationship that the preferences of individual patients should be the determining factor in any decisions that have to be made about their access to particular treatments. Suppose that patients have actively participated in discussions about their clinical need and treatment options. Any further *rationing* decisions about whether or not they receive specific treatments or the order in which they do so should be determined only by procedural rules of the sort that have been outlined for optimising fairness. These will trump the understandable, though sometimes irrational, concern with self interest which sustained illness often brings about.

In such circumstances, patients may well demand resources that they do not need or to which their level of need does not entitle them at that point in time. Scarce clinical resources should never be employed just because patients—or their relatives—want them. If a decision is to be made to withhold health care that patients and relatives believe will be of benefit, clinical teams must be very sure that their clinical assessment of futility is accurate or their procedural justification is morally coherent for providing treatment at a later date. Here, the participation—and sometimes protestations—of their patients may be crucial for making a correct decision. Equally, however, part of the duty of care includes sensitive and coherent explanations of why treatment is not being offered (or discontinued) and why it is members of the clinical team, rather than the patient, who have ultimate responsibility for this decision.

Conclusion

The moral foundations of the NHS do not depend on a majority vote or individual preference for their moral coherence. Their justification starts and finishes with the quality of moral arguments employed, along with the empirical evidence referred to in such argument. It follows that principles of equality and fairness in the rationing of health care should not be open to change on any other basis. It is not morally acceptable that, in some parts of the country but not others, a minority of patients in serious need are denied access to particular treatments. Such local discrimination should not be allowed. Some rights must be protected from collective and individual arbitrariness. The right of access to appropriate health on the basis of equal need is one of them.

1 New B. The rationing agenda in the NHS. *BMJ* 1996;**312**:1593-601.
2 NHS Management Executive. *Local voices: The views of local people in purchasing*. London: HMSO, 1992.
3 Farrell C, Gilbert H. *Health care partnerships*. London: King's Fund, 1996.
4 Cooper L, Coote A, Davis A, Jackson C. *Voices off: tackling the democratic deficit in health*. London: IPPR, 1995.

5 Gutmann A. *Liberal equality.* Cambridge: Cambridge University Press, 1980.
6 Held D. *Models of democracy.* Oxford: Polity, 1996.
7 McLean I. Forms of representation and systems of voting. In: Held D, ed. *Political theory today.* Oxford, Polity, 1991.
8 Stewart J. *Further innovation in democratic practice.* Birmingham: Institute of Local Government Studies, University of Birmingham, 1996.
9 Stewart J, Kendall E, Coote A. *Citizen juries.* London: Institute for Public Policy Research; 1994.
10 Doyal L, Gough I. *A theory of human need.* London: Macmillan, 1991.
11 Pfeffer N, Pollock A. Public opinion and the NHS. *BMJ* 1993;**307**:750–75.
12 Boyle S, Dixon J, Harrison A. Financial meltdown for the NHS? *BMJ* 1996;**312**:1432–3.
13 Dixon J, Harrison A. Funding the NHS—A little local difficulty? *BMJ* 1997;**314**:216–19.
14 Crail M. How the tables have turned. *Health Services J* 1995;16 February:14–15.
15 Klein R, Day P, Redmayne S. *Managing scarcity—priority setting and rationing in the National Health Service.* Buckingham: Open University Press, 1996.
16 Kennedy I. "What is a medical decision". In: Kennedy I ed. *Treat me right: Essays in medical law and ethics.* Oxford: Clarendon Press, 1988:19–31.
17 Bowie C, Richardson A, Sykes W. Consulting the public about health service priorities. *BMJ* 1995;**311**:1155–8.
18 Stewart J, Honigsbaum F, Richards J, Lockett T. *Priority setting in action—purchasing dilemmas.* Birmingham: Health Services Management Centre, 1995.
19 Heginbotham C. Health care priority setting: a survey of doctors, managers, and the general public. In: *Rationing in action.* London: BMJ Publishing Group 1993.
20 Bowling A. Health care rationing: the public's debate. *BMJ* 1996;**312**:670–7.
21 Jacobson B, Bowling A. Involving the public: practical and ethical issues. In: Maxwell R, ed. *Rationing health care.* London: Churchill Livingstone, 1995:869–75.
22 Plant R. Citizenship and rights. In: Milligan D, Miller W, eds. *Liberalism, citizenship and autonomy.* Aldershot: Avebury, 1992:108–33.
23 Dworkin R. Will Clinton's plan be fair? *New York Review of Books* 1994:January 13:20–5.
24 Redmayne S. *Reshaping the NHS: strategies and priorities and resource allocation.* Birmingham: National Association of Health Authorities and Trusts, 1995.
25 Stacey M. *The sociology of health and healing.* London: Unwin Hyman, 1988.
26 Doyal L. Needs, rights, and equity: moral quality in health care rationing. *Quality in Health Care* 1995;**4**:273–83.
27 Lenaghan J. *Rationing and rights in health care.* London: Institute for Public Policy Research, 1996.
28 Williams G, Popay J. *Researching the people's health: dilemmas and opportunities for social scientists in researching the people's health.* London: Routledge, 1994.
29 Pfeffer N, Coote A. *Is quality good for you?* London: Institute for Public Policy Research, 1991.
30 Percy-Smith J, Sanderson I. *Understanding local needs.* London: Institute for Public Policy Research, 1992.
31 Doyal L. Need for moral audit in evaluating quality in health care. *Quality in Health Care* 1992;**1**:178-83.
32 Davis H, Fallowfield L eds. Counselling and communication in health care. Chichester: John Wiley, 1991:3–22.

Section 2:
"Action"

12 The New Zealand priority criteria project

DAVID C HADORN, ANDREW C HOLMES

Part 1: Overview

In this chapter we describe a national project, sponsored jointly by New Zealand's National Advisory Committee on Health and Disability and the four regional health authorities, to develop standardised priority assessment criteria for elective surgical procedures. Under the auspices of this project, criteria were developed for cataract extraction, coronary artery bypass graft surgery, hip and knee replacement, cholecystectomy, and tympanostomy tubes for otitis media with effusion. These criteria are used (1) to assess patients' relative priority for surgery, (2) to ensure consistency and transparency in the provision of surgical services across New Zealand, and (3) to provide a basis for describing the kinds of patients who will or will not receive surgery under various possible levels of funding.

New Zealand health reforms

As part of a sweeping overhaul of its economy and social structure, New Zealand implemented major reforms of its healthcare system in 1992 (see box).[1] These reforms can be viewed as a response to the imperatives described by Relman in his 1988 editorial in the *New England Journal of Medicine* announcing the arrival of the era of assessment and accountability in health care.[2] Relman called for a "revolution" in how health care is provided and paid for, endorsing a proposal put forth by Elwood in the same journal just a few months earlier. Elwood described the problem like this:

Too often, payers, physicians, and health care executives do not share common insights into the life of the patient. We acknowledge that our common interest is the patient, but we represent that interest from such

183

divergent, even conflicting, viewpoints that everyone loses perspective. As a result, the health care system has become an organism guided by misguided choices; it is unstable, confused, and desperately in need of a central nervous system that can help it cope with the complexities of modern medicine.[3]

The New Zealand health reforms represent an effort to provide such a central nervous system. Elwood proposed that the healthcare system should routinely collect detailed clinical information concerning (1) the quantity and kinds of services provided, (2) the numbers and kinds of patients receiving those services, and (3) the outcomes experienced by those patients. Recognition of the need for such assessment data and for better channels of communication constituted a major rationale for the restructuring. At the same time, the contract mechanism was seen as a useful method for ensuring provider accountability.

National health committee

A major component of the legislation under which the healthcare system was restructured was the creation of a National Advisory Committee on Core Health and Disability Support Services, since renamed the National Advisory Committee on Health and Disability—and known as the National Health Committee. This committee is charged with providing independent advice to the Minister of Health (independent, in particular, of the Ministry of Health) concerning the "kinds, and relative priorities, of public health services, personal health services, and disability services that should, in the committee's opinion, be publicly funded".[4]

Early in its tenure the National Health Committee came under considerable pressure to develop a relatively simple list of services depicting what was in or out of the "core" of services that would be publicly funded.

New Zealand health reforms

- Fourteen area health boards were replaced with four regional health authorities, which purchase publicly funded health and disability services. The National Advisory Committee on Health and Disability was created to advise the Minister of Health on the kinds of services to be purchased with public funds—and their priority.
- The Ministry of Health (formerly Department of Health) is responsible for macro policy making and funding. Inpatient services are provided predominantly by crown health enterprises (hospitals and affiliated institutions), which are managed as businesses and are state owned.
- A complete split exists in funding, purchasing, and provision of services.

Project methods

- A summary of the relevant literature was prepared by project staff.
- Professional advisory groups were constituted for each procedure, consisting of two or three specialists and surgeons from each of the four regions, and two general practitioners.
- A two stage Delphi process preceding each professional advisory group meeting was open to all relevant specialists and surgeons in New Zealand (about 20–30 clinicians participated for each procedure, not counting members of the professional advisory groups).
- Criteria were selected and initial weights agreed at meetings of the professional advisory groups. The draft criteria were pilot tested and their weights recalibrated based on the results.

From the outset, however, the Committee has taken a different approach. It has preferred to define eligibility for services in terms of clinical practice guidelines or explicit assessment criteria which depict the circumstances under which patients are likely to derive substantial health benefit from those services, bearing in mind competing claims on resources. Thus, for example, patients could reasonably expect to receive coronary bypass graft surgery at the taxpayer's expense if (and only if) their clinical circumstances were commensurate with a likelihood of substantial benefit from that procedure.

The waiting list problem

Long waiting lists for elective surgery have been a nagging issue that long predated the formation of the Ministry, Regional Health Authorities, and the National Health Committee. Based on one of its early commissioned reports,[5] the National Health Committee recommended that surgical services should move away from a system of waiting lists and towards a system of specific booking times, so that patients would know (within reasonable limits) when they would receive their operation. In addition, the Committee called for greater transparency and consistency in the process used to decide priority for elective surgery.[6]

The Minister, the Ministry, and the Regional Health Authorities accepted the National Health Committee's advice, including the replacement of waiting lists with booking systems. As a step towards realising this goal, the Regional Health Authorities and National Health Committee cosponsored a national project to put in place the tools needed to assess the extent of patients' overall priority or urgency for surgery. These priority criteria would reflect primarily the benefit expected from surgery. Priority would generally be given to patients with the greatest likely benefit.

Thus, the ethical framework under which the project was conducted was largely utilitarian in nature, with the principal goal being to achieve the maximum possible health gain with the available funds. The National Health Committee had formally embraced the philosophy of maximising expected benefit in one of its early reports.[6]

The national priority criteria project

A six member project steering group was constituted, consisting of representatives of the National Health Committee (DCH and ACH) and the surgical services managers of the four Regional Health Authorities. Ministry of Health officials were briefed regularly but were not members of the steering group. The stated objective of the project was:

To develop national criteria for assessing the priority which should be given to patients for medical and surgical procedures. .... The national priority criteria will serve the following purposes:
(1) To ensure that the process used to define priority is fair and consistent across New Zealand.
(2) To permit the assessment and comparison of need, case mix, and severity.
(3) To assist the regional health authorities in developing new booking strategies, including target booking times for patients with defined levels of priority.
(4) To permit comparison of waiting times across regional health authorities.
(5) To ensure that social values are integrated into the decision making process in an appropriate and transparent manner.
(6) To provide the framework for the National Health Committee to define maximum acceptable waiting times for patients with defined levels of priority, as well as core levels of each service.
(7) To make possible national studies on the health outcomes experienced by patients who do or do not receive the services.

The box on page 185 summarises the approach taken to develop the criteria.

Progress to date

Five sets of standardised assessment criteria were developed for elective surgical procedures under the auspices of the project. Numerical scores

186

were assigned to each of the multiple levels of severity on each criterion; relevant scores on each criterion were added together to form a total score. These multiple factor, additive systems are known as linear models. Such models are well known to outperform unaided clinical judgment on a wide variety of diagnostic and predictive tasks.[7-9]

The procedures covered are (in order of development):

(1) Cataract extraction
(2) Coronary artery bypass graft surgery
(3) Hip and knee replacement
(4) Cholecystectomy
(5) Tympanostomy tubes for otitis media with effusion.

Table 12.1 shows the criteria for cataract extraction and table 12.2 those for hip and knee replacement. All criteria were subject to a pilot study to assess the extent of correspondence between the total priority score and global clinical judgments of urgency. A description of the development of the criteria for coronary artery bypass grafting together with their pilot study are described in part 2 of this chapter. Additional information on the pilot studies is available on the *BMJ*'s Internet web site (www.bmj.com).

Social factors considered in setting priorities

As well as clinical criteria, several social factors were discussed during the course of this project and, to some extent, incorporated within the priority criteria. The most important of these were (1) age, (2) work status, (3) whether patients were caring for dependants or threatened with the loss of their own independence, and (4) time spent on the waiting list.

Age

There was substantial disagreement among project participants about the appropriate role of patients' age in assessing the expected benefit from surgery. From a practical perspective, many participants considered age to be a roughly reliable guide to the overall extent of co-morbidity experienced by patients, which in turn affects the extent of benefit that can be expected from surgery. Others were, however, concerned that, even if this is true on average, use of age as a factor in deciding priority for surgery could result in denying services to many elderly patients who would benefit as much as (or more than) younger patients. In the end, age was incorporated in just one set of criteria: those for coronary artery bypass graft surgery. The rationale for its inclusion here was that this type of surgery has direct implications for life expectancy as well as quality of life, whereas the other

Table 12.1   Priority criteria for cataract surgery (maximum score 100)

Clinical features							Score
Visual acuity	6/9 or better	6/12	6/18	6/24	6/36	6/60	Count fingers/hand movements
6/9 or better	0	1	2	3	4	5	6
6/12		7	8	9	10	11	12
6/18			14	15	16	17	18
6/24				21	22	23	24
6/36					28	29	30
6/60						35	36
Count fingers/hand movements							40

Glare	
None	0
Mild–moderate	5
Severe	10

Ocular co-morbidity (eg age-related macular degeneration, chronic simple glaucoma)	
None	0
Mild–moderate	5
Severe	10

Ability to work, care for dependants, or work independently	
Not threatened or not applicable	0
Not threatened but more difficult	2
Threatened but not immediately	6
Immediately threatened	15

Extent of impairment in visual function (eg reading, recognising faces, see steps or kerbs, watching TV, driving, and reading traffic signs)	
None	0
Mild	5
Moderate	10
Severe	20

Other substantial disability (eg hearing loss, uses wheelchair)	
No	0
Yes	5

Total score	

surgical procedures directly affect only quality of life. The professional advisory group on coronary artery bypass grafting believed that life prolongation becomes progressively less important for elderly patients compared with the importance of quality of life. Accordingly, the group developed a formula to adjust downward, beginning at age 70, the weights assigned to variables associated with improvements in life expectancy (see *BMJ* web site for details.)

Table 12.2   Priority criteria for major joint replacement (maximum score 100)

Clinical features	Score
Pain (40%)	
Degree (patient must be on maximum medical therapy at time of rating):	
None	0
Mild: slight or occasional pain; patient has not altered patterns of activity or work	4
Mild–moderate: moderate or frequent pain; patient has not altered patterns of activity or work	6
Moderate: patient is active but has had to modify or give up some activities because of pain	9
Moderate–severe: fairly severe pain with substantially limited activities	14
Severe: major pain and serious limitations	20
Occurrence:	
None or with first steps only	0
Only after long walks (30 minuts)	4
With all walking, mostly day pain	10
Significant, regular night pain	20
Functional activity (20%)	
Time walked:	
Unlimited	0
31–60 minutes (eg longer shopping trips to mall)	2
11–30 minutes (eg gardening, grocery shopping)	4
2–10 minutes (eg trip to letter box)	6
<2 minutes or indoors only (more or less house bound)	8
Unable to walk	10
Other functional limitations (eg putting on shoes, managing stairs, sitting to standing, sexual activity, recreation or hobbies, walking aids needed):	
None	0
Mild	2
Moderate	4
Severe	10
Movement and deformity (20%)	
Pain on examination (overall results are both active and passive range of motion):	
None	0
Mild	2
Moderate	5
Severe	10
Other abnormal findings (limited to orthopaedic problems eg reduced range of motion, deformity, limp, instability, progressive x ray findings):	
None	0
Mild	2
Moderate	5
Severe	10
Other factors (20%)	
Multiple joint disease:	
No, single joint	0
Yes, each affected joint mild: moderate in severity	4
Yes, severe involvement (eg severe rheumatoid arthritis)	10
Ability to work, give care to dependants, live independently (difficulty must be related to affected joint):	
Not threatened or difficult	70
Not threatened but more difficult	4
Threatened but not immediately	6
Immediately threatened	10
Total score	

Threat to independence, care of dependants, ability to work

During the process of identifying the factors currently used by clinicians to make judgments of expected benefit, project participants acknowledged that clinicians take into account whether (and to what extent) patients' clinical conditions threaten their ability to work, care for dependants, and live independently. Substantial discussion was held on this topic at each professional advisory group meeting, with clinicians generally agreeing that these factors should be represented as priority criteria. Nevertheless, a certain degree of misgiving was usually noted about incorporating these social factors. To address this issue, the National Health Committee sponsored two public hearings, one on each major island, specifically devoted to discussing the appropriateness of including these factors in the assessment of urgency and priority for elective surgery. A stratified random sample of the public in each community and patients with the relevant conditions were recruited to provide their perspectives. Clinicians from the local area and members of the professional advisory groups also attended. Although no definitive resolution was achieved, the results of the hearings were regarded by observers from the National Health Committee and Regional Health Authorities as supporting the inclusion of these factors, provided they are given relatively little weight compared with clinical factors.

Time spent on waiting list

The length of time spent waiting for the procedure also proved a contentious and difficult issue. Many clinicians favoured inclusion of such a factor on grounds that the "simple act of waiting" should warrant some consideration. However, this concern was balanced by the fact that, if waiting time were incorporated, the inevitable result would be that in many cases less impaired patients would be operated on before more impaired patients. In the end, "time spent waiting" was excluded from the criteria, mainly because the principal tenet of the criteria is that they reflect the degree of clinical (and social) probable benefit associated with the clinical condition, not time spent waiting.

Minister of Health's announcement

On 8 May 1996 the Minister of Health, Jenny Shipley, announced the creation of a new NZ$130m (£57m; US$90m) fund with the express purpose of reducing waiting times and clearing waiting lists. Access to the funds is contingent on the use of explicit clinical priority criteria, such as, but not limited to, those developed during this project.

Professional and public response is generally positive

Response to the new waiting list initiative has been generally positive. In particular, the response from doctors has been largely one of relief that thousands of patients on waiting lists will now be provided with surgery who would not have received it without these new funds. News coverage has also been generally favourable. The capital's *Dominion* described the move as another "welcome step toward reducing waiting lists for non–urgent surgery in a responsible way, instead of resorting to the bad old practice of throwing money at a problem and hoping for the best. . . . The new system is designed to ensure that people with the biggest need and greatest potential benefit will have their surgery first, that the same rules apply throughout New Zealand. . . . All this is light years ahead of rationing surgery by making people wait indefinitely for it, and with marked regional variations".[10]

In part 2 we describe in more detail our experience developing, testing, and implementing the priority criteria for coronary artery bypass graft surgery.

Acknowledgments

We thank the many clinicians who participated in this project without whose support this project could not have been completed successfully.

1 Ashton T. From evolution to revolution: restructuring the New Zealand health system. *Health Care Analysis* 1993;**1**:57–62.
2 Relman AS. Assessment and accountability: the third revolution in medical care. *N Engl J Med* 1988;**319**:1220–2.
3 Elwood PM. Outcomes management: a technology of patient experience. *N Engl J Med* 1988;**318**:1549–56.
4 Health and Disability Act 1993, as amended 1995; Sec 8, par 2, p5.
5 Fraser G, Alley P, Morris R. *Waiting lists and waiting times: their nature and management.* Wellington: National Advisory Committee on Core Health and Disability Support Services, 1993.
6 National Advisory Committee on Core Health and Disability Support Services. *Second annual report.* Wellington: National Advisory Committee on Core Health and Disability Support Services, 1993.
7 Dawes RM, Corrigan B. Linear models in decision making. *Psychol Bull* 1974;**81**:95–106.
8 Meehl PK. *Clinical versus statistical prediction: a theoretical analysis and a review of the evidence.* Minneapolis: University of Minnesota Press, 1954.
9 Tversky A, Kahneman D. *Judgment under uncertainty: heuristics and biases.* Cambridge: Cambridge University Press, 1982.
10 Editorial. *Dominion.* 1996;10 May:8.

Part 2: Coronary artery bypass graft surgery

This section discusses several issues arising from the priority criteria project in the context of the criteria developed for coronary artery bypass surgery. We describe the process of developing criteria, including the results of a pilot test, and discuss how the results of a clinical audit of all patients on New Zealand's waiting lists for coronary artery bypass grafting were used to estimate the cost of providing surgery to patients down to each of several possible clinical thresholds. A new government initiative to clear waiting lists is described which requires use of explicit criteria such as those developed in this project. We discuss how cardiologists and cardiac surgeons agreed to accept a specific numerical threshold as indicative of reasonable levels of service provision. Finally, we describe how the criteria were used to identify and describe the kinds of patients who would or would not receive coronary artery bypass surgery at defined levels of public funding.

Background

Development of the criteria for coronary artery bypass grafting as part of the priority criteria project followed similar work reported by clinicians at Greenlane Hospital in Auckland,[1] which itself had been motivated by earlier work on waiting lists sponsored by the National Health Committee on Health and Disability.[2,3] The results of the Greenlane study, which used a method based on the rating system developed by Naylor and co–workers,[4] had called into question the extent to which quantitative measures could capture clinicians' overall judgments of priority and probable benefit. Nevertheless, the Greenlane investigators, all of whom were also members of our professional advisory group on coronary artery bypass grafting, agreed it was important to continue the effort to develop such criteria.

Clinicians' reactions to the project

In general clinicians in New Zealand were very interested in the project and willing to participate despite tight timetables and nominal reimbursement. Almost all clinicians who were nominated by Regional Health Authorities agreed to serve as professional advisory group members, and 20–30 additional clinicians from around the country took time to provide often extensive responses to requests for comments on each

192

procedure. As described in part 1, all relevant specialists and surgeons were invited to provide comments as part of a modified Delphi process.

As might be expected, clinicians had mixed views on the project. The most commonly expressed concern was that the Government or the Regional Health Authorities would use the criteria to specify arbitrary numerical cut off points below which surgery would not be funded. In the minds of many clinicians the real problem was that the level of funding for surgical services was inadequate. Developing a priority system in the context of such scarcity would be like "rearranging the deck chairs on the Titanic", as one commentator put it. Similarly, a member of the professional advisory group for coronary artery bypass grafting wrote, "If the available surgical resource is inadequate, it is not possible to produce a workable numerical system of prioritisation for patients in need of coronary artery surgery".

Despite these concerns physicians and surgeons from around New Zealand cooperated with this project to a very substantial extent. Two principal reasons for this cooperation were identified. First, clinicians almost universally acknowledged that decisions about urgency and priority were made inconsistently. Often, the "squeaky wheel would get the grease", and more deserving but uncomplaining patients would be disadvantaged. One cardiologist put it like this:

> Manipulation by referring doctors, friends in high places, MP letters, or just persistent nagging, and just slight exaggeration of symptoms, is rampant, and the poor benign patient simply sits on the list and is leap frogged. I support any system which will provide fair, humane, and prognostic order of surgery.

The second major reason for clinicians' cooperation in this project was their wish to develop an objective measure of symptoms and functional status that policy makers could understand. Participating clinicians viewed the development of standardised assessment criteria as having the potential to provide additional, more comprehensible, and possibly dramatic information concerning the extent of "unmet need".

Development of criteria for coronary artery bypass grafting

The priority criteria for coronary artery bypass grafting were developed by a professional advisory group consisting of seven cardiologists, four cardiac surgeons, one physician, and two general practitioners. These individuals were nominated by the four Regional Health Authorities and

193

by the Royal New Zealand College of General Practitioners. Selection of the criteria followed an iterative modified Delphi consensus process, including consideration of written comments received from an additional 25 cardiologists and surgeons from around New Zealand (see part 1).

As described in part 1, the priority criteria represent the clinical factors—for example, the extent of coronary artery obstruction—that have been shown, or are considered, to be associated with the degree of benefit obtained from the procedure. Numerical scores (or weights) are assigned to each of multiple levels of severity on each criterion; relevant scores on each criterion are then added together to form a total score. This score is considered indicative of the overall degree of benefit expected from surgery (see table 12.3).

In selecting priority criteria for coronary artery bypass grafting the professional advisory group was able to rely to a much greater extent on published outcome studies than were the advisory groups for the other procedures (cataract surgery, hip and knee replacement, cholecystectomy, and tympanostomy tubes for otitis media with effusion. For example, a table listing the various possible degrees of coronary artery obstruction was adopted without significant change from a then newly published analysis of 10 years' experience with coronary artery bypass grafting by Duke University investigators.[5] The initial weights assigned to these degrees of obstruction were taken directly from this published report, although recalibrated to accommodate the 100 point maximum adopted for each set of criteria.

Weights were assigned to the remaining factors based on additional information in this report and from a meta–analysis of outcomes of coronary artery bypass grafting published during this process.[6] It was agreed that these initial weights would be revised as appropriate based on the results of a pilot study. As described in part 1, both a "social factor" and an age adjustment factor were incorporated into the clinical criteria to reflect both common clinical practice and the balance of social values, as gleaned by the national health committee via public meetings and consultation.

Pilot study

A formal pilot study was conducted of each set of criteria. Details of the methods and results of these studies are available on the *BMJ*'s worldwide web site (www.bmj.com). We briefly describe the coronary artery bypass grafting criteria pilot study here.

A total of 260 patients was assessed during the study. Of these, 133 patients were evaluated at Greenlane Hospital (Auckland), 119 at Dunedin Hospital, and eight at Waikato Hospital (Hamilton). Although patients

Table 12.3 Priority criteria for coronary artery bypass surgery (maximum score 100)

Clinical feature	Score
Degree of coronary artery obstruction (% diameter occluded)	
No coronary artery disease (≥50%)	0
One vessel disease (50–74%)	8
Disease of more than one vessel (50–74%)	9
One vessel disease (75%)	9
One vessel disease (≥90%)	14
Two vessel disease (50–89%)	15
Two vessel disease (both ≥90%)	15
One vessel disease (≥90%) proximal left anterior descending artery	19
Two vessel disease (≥90%) left anterior descending artery	19
Two vessel disease (≥90%) proximal left anterior descending artery	19
Three vessel disease	19
Three vessel disease (≥90%) in at least one	19
Three vessel disease (75%) proximal left anterior descending artery	19
Three vessel disease (≥90%) proximal left anterior descending artery	27
Left main (50%)	27
Left main (75%)	32
Left main (≥90%)	36
Angina (Canadian Cardiovascular Society criteria: class of angina after appropriate treatment)	
Class I: angina on strenuous exertion	1
Class II: angina on walking or climbing stairs rapidly	2
Class III: angina on walking one or two level blocks	8
Class IV A: unstable angina, rest pain	18
Class IV B: unstable angina on oral treatment, in hospital. Symptoms improved on treatment but angina with minimal provocation	22
Class IV C: in hospital on intravenous heparin or glycery trinitrate	26
Exercise stress test (Bruce protocol*)	
Negative	0
Mildly positive	8
Positive	12
Very positive	22
Ability to work, care for dependants, or live independently	
Not threatened but more difficult	1
Threatened but not immediately	5
Immediately threatened	16

* Very positive: ≥2 mm ST depression ± angina in stage I, fall in blood pressure >15 mm HG in stages I–II, ventricular tachycardia or fibrillation in stages I–II, or unsafe to perform test; Positive: any of the above criteria but patient not on optimal treatment or inability to progress beyond stage II for other reasons; Mildly positive: test stopped at stage III; Negative: none of the above or test stopped at stage IV.

were enrolled more or less consecutively during the study period, the sample should be considered a convenience sample.

Total priority scores were calculated for each patient by adding the weights assigned to various factors at the appropriate levels. In addition, physicians were asked to estimate what a "reasonable waiting time" (in

Table 12.4   The estimated cost of providing surgery on a steady state basis to patients at or above each of various possible clinical thresholds, highlighting the level of current funding (threshold 35 points)

No. of operations per week	No. of operations per year	Priority threshold	Estimated cost (NZ$)*
17	884	44	14 500 000
18	936	42	15 400 000
19	988	40	16 300 000
20	1040	39	17 200 000
21	1092	37	18 100 000
22	1144	35	19 000 000
23	1196	34	19 900 000
24	1248	32	20 700 000
25	1300	31	21 600 000
26	1352	29	22 500 000
27	1404	27	23 400 000
28	1456	25	24 300 000
29	1508	21	25 200 000
30	1560	7	26 000 000

* Based on unit costs of NZ$17 000 per elective operation, NZ$22 000 per acute operation (10 per week). 1NZ$ = £0·44, US$0·70.

days) would be for each patient, considering an "adequately, not infinitely funded service" and "keeping in mind competing claims for resources both within and outside the health sector". Reasonable waiting time, which was considered indicative of likely benefit, was used as the outcome (dependent) variable in our analyses. Alternative dependent variables could have been used, such as clinicians' global assessment of expected benefit on a scale of 0–100. It is unclear whether the results of our analysis would have differed substantially had an alternative dependent variable been used.

Regression analysis was used to determine the set of criteria weights resulting in the highest degree of correlation between priority scores and clinicians' judgments of reasonable waiting times. Slight modifications were then made in a few weights based on clinical judgment. The final criteria and weights (table 12.3) correlated quite closely with estimates of reasonable waiting time, with a statistical test of correspondence (coefficient of variation, or R^2) of 0·62 (perfect correlation would score 1·0, no correlation would score 0).

Based on the results of the pilot test we calculated the approximate cost of providing surgery to patients who present for coronary artery bypass grafting in New Zealand on a steady state basis—that is, assuming that a separate (and separately funded) initiative were used to clear the waiting lists (as discussed below). Table 12.4 shows the estimated cost of providing surgery to patients at or above each of various possible clinical thresholds.

Table 12.5   Summary of costs for performing coronary artery bypass grafting on 662 patients on New Zealand's waiting lists

Priority score threshold	Proportion operated on	No. of patients operated on	Cost (NZ$)*
65	0·02	12	200 000
60	0·04	25	430 000
55	0·08	56	950 000
50	0·14	94	1 600 000
45	0·24	157	2 700 000
40	0·36	237	4 000 000
35	0·51	337	5 700 000
30	0·69	454	7 700 000
25	0·87	574	9 800 000
20	0·95	626	10 600 000
15	0·99	655	11 100 000
10	1·00	660	11 200 000
5	1·00	661	11 200 000
0	1·00	662	11 300 000

* Based on a unit cost of NZ$17 000 per operation. 1 NZ$ = £0·44, US$0·70.

On current funding levels we estimate that coronary artery bypass grafting can be provided to patients scoring 35 points or higher.

Audit of waiting lists for coronary artery bypass grafting

Following development, testing, and revision of the criteria for coronary artery bypass grafting a clinical audit was conducted of all patients on New Zealand's waiting lists for coronary artery bypass grafting using the revised criteria. A single, experienced, independent nurse reviewer examined the clinical records of all 662 patients on the four regional waiting lists and abstracted from those records the data required for calculating priority scores. Standardised abstraction forms and coding protocols were developed to provide additional assurance of comparability across centres.

The observed distribution of priority scores for patients on waiting lists for coronary artery bypass grafting in New Zealand was roughly normal (fig 12.1).

Based on this distribution, we calculated the cost of providing coronary artery bypass grafting surgery to all patients on current public waiting lists at or above specified thresholds of clinical priority (table 12.5). These estimates were derived using various assumptions concerning the unit cost

197

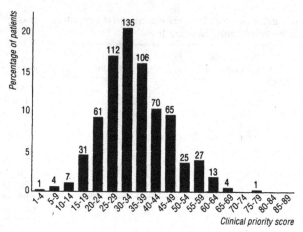

Clinical priority score

Fig. 12.1 Distribution of priority scores for coronary artery bypass grafting among 662 patients waiting for the operation in New Zealand. Numbers of patients are given above each bar

of coronary artery bypass grafting and the proportion of patients on lists who would no longer benefit from surgery.

Describing kinds of patients

The priority criteria used in this project lend themselves to the purpose of providing a "common insight into the life of the patient". In the case of coronary artery bypass grafting, patients were described by reference to five point bands on the scale of clinical priority. Within each band, patients were ordered on each variable and the median values of each variable identified. The collection of median values on all four variables was used to describe the "average patient" within each five point band. Table 12.6 depicts the results of this process.

For purposes of communicating more directly to politicians, policy makers, and the public a greater degree of descriptive richness was considered necessary. For this reason, the range of priority scores was divided into three levels and the median values of patients within each level identified. Descriptions based on these values were constructed using the operational definitions of angina (see table 12.3) together with estimates of the likely implications of coronary artery bypass grafting surgery on life expectancy. These estimates were based on an examination of a recent meta-analysis.[6] The resulting descriptions are presented in the box. These descriptions were deemed by most observers to be valid and effective

198

Table 12.6 Median levels of each clinical variable within each 5 point priority score band for coronary artery bypass grafting, April 1996

Priority score	No.	Coronary artery disease	Angina	Exercise stress test	Ability	Age (years)
10–14	6	One vessel disease (75%)	Class II	Negative	Not threatened	67·5
15–19	29	Two vessel disease (50–94%)	Class II	Negative	Not threatened	66·9
20–24	54	Three vessel disease	Class II	Mildly positive	Not threatened	64·6
25–29	126	Three vessel disease	Class II	Mildly positive	Not threatened	63·2
30–34	123	Three vessel disease ($\geq$95%) in at least 1	Class II	Positive	Not threatened	62·8
35–39	112	Three vessel disease ($\geq$95%) in at least 1	Class III	Positive	Threatened but not immediately	62·0
40–44	89	Three vessel disease (75%) proximal left anterior descending artery	Class II	Positive	Threatened but not immediately	59·9
45–49	68	Three vessel disease (75%) proximal left anterior descending artery	Class III	Positive	Immediately threatened	63·2
50–54	42	Three vessel disease (75%) proximal left anterior descending artery	Class III	Very positive	Immediately threatened	59·6
55–59	35	Three vessel disease ($\geq$95%) proximal left anterior descending artery	Class III	Very positive	Immediately threatened	60·4
60–64	15	Three vessel disease ($\geq$95%) proximal left anterior descending artery	Class III	Very positive	Immediately threatened	64·8
65–69	8	Three vessel disease (75%) proximal left anterior descending artery	Class IV A	Very positive	Immediately threatened	59·6

descriptions of patient severity with which to communicate to the public and policy makers.

Specification of clinically desirable threshold

As described in part 1, on 8 May 1996 the Minister of Health announced the creation of a NZ$130m fund to be used for clearing surgical waiting lists and replacing them with booking systems. On that same day the

---

Descriptions of average patient at each of three levels of priority score

- Patients with a score of 55 or more have considerably reduced quality of life due to chest pain and breathlessness on almost any physical activity and a reduction in life expectancy of perhaps 1–2 years in the absence of surgery.
- Patients with scores of 35–54 experience much reduced quality of life, mainly through pain on exertion, such as walking one or two blocks, as well as moderately (8–12 months) reduced life expectancy in the absence of surgery.
- Patients with scores of 25–34 points experience intermittent pain or breathlessness when undertaking such activities as walking or climbing stairs rapidly and experience a modest reduction in life expectancy (4–8 months) in the absence of surgery.

Minister also launched a meeting attended by cardiologists, cardiac surgeons, and representatives of the Ministry of Health, National Health Committee, and Regional Health Authorities.

The results of the audit just described were presented at that meeting. The clinicians accepted the results of the audit and, after discussion, agreed that a clinical threshold of 25 points before considering coronary artery bypass grafting was reasonable given the degree of benefit expected and competing claims on resources. Whether public funding would be sufficient to operate on all patients above this threshold was recognised by all participants to be a separate, societal question. Indeed, at the meeting the Minister agreed to be held accountable for any gap between what is clinically desirable and what is financially sustainable, reasoning that appropriate funding levels must take into account competing claims on resources—adjudication of which is ultimately up to society to resolve through democratic processes.

As noted earlier, preliminary estimates indicate that current funding levels will permit surgery to be offered to patients scoring at or above 35 points. As such, there is an apparent 10 point gap between what is clinically preferred and what can be afforded. We believe that the ability to quantify this gap, even if imperfectly, represents a major advantage of the general approach described in this article.

The acceptance by clinicians of a quantitative threshold for surgery, based on priority criteria, represents a key development in the transition within New Zealand from waiting lists to booking systems. Such explicit

200

acceptance by clinicians of the inevitability of limits is vital to the success of any attempt to distribute healthcare dollars more equitably. On balance, we believe the experiences described in this article are an important step towards the goal of a fair, transparent, and evidence based allocation policy.

Acknowledgments

We thank our professional advisory group for their support and help, especially Dr Trevor Agnew and Mr Richard Bunton; Annmarie Banchy for her excellent work in conducting the national audit of coronary artery bypass graft waiting lists; and Paul O'Connor for performing the statistical analysis.

1 Agnew TM, Whitlock RML, Neutze JM, Kerr AR. Waiting lists for coronary artery bypass surgery: can they be better organised? *N Z Med J* 1994;107:211–5.
2 National Advisory Committee on Core Health and Disability Support Services. *Second annual report*. Wellington: National Advisory Committee on Core Health and Disability Support Services, 1993.
3 Fraser G, Alley P, Morris R. *Waiting lists and waiting times: their nature and management.* Wellington: National Advisory Committee on Core Health and Disability Support Services, 1993.
4 Naylor CD, Baigre RS, Goldman BS, Basinski A. Assessment of priority for coronary revascularisation procedures. *Lancet* 1990;335:1070–3.
5 Mark DB, Nelson CL, Califf RM, Harrell FE, Lee KL, Jones RH, *et al.* Continuing evolution of therapy for coronary artery disease. *Circulation* 1994;89:2015–25.
6 Yusuf S, Zucker D, Peduzzi P, Fisher LD, Takaro T, Kennedy JW, *et al.* Effect of coronary artery bypass graft surgery on survival: overview of 10–year results from randomised trials by the Coronary Artery Bypass Graft Surgery Trialists Collaboration. *Lancet* 1994;344: 563–70.
7 Elwood PM. Outcomes management: a technology of patient experience. *N Engl J Med* 1988;318:1549–56.

13 Setting priorities: can Britain learn from Sweden?

MARTIN McKEE, JOSEP FIGUERAS

Throughout the industrialised world there is concern about the apparent mismatch between demand for health care and the resources that governments are prepared to commit to meet it. The reasons are complex, the effects vary between nations, and most of the reasons are poorly understood, although they include the effects of ageing populations, the introduction of new technology, and rising public expectations. The responses by countries have also varied widely, depending on factors such as the relative power of governments, the medical profession, insurance companies, and national pharmaceutical industries.

Five possible approaches to the mismatch between demands and resources exist: increasing resources either from government revenues or from individuals; controlling either demand (through cost sharing) or supply of services; withdrawing funding from services that are ineffective or where there is a cheaper alternative; increasing the efficiency of service provision; or creating a mechanism explicitly to identify health care priorities.[1] With the possible exception of controls on supply, using capital and personnel ceilings or global budgets, as in the UK and Germany, there is little evidence that the first four have been successful in controlling the apparently inexorable rise in health care expenditure. Some, however, such as reducing ineffective care, have been difficult to implement. Consequently, there is growing interest in the fifth—explicitly trying to define what types of health care might no longer be provided from public resources. In the UK this approach has been variously described as rationing or priority setting, the choice of term partially reflecting the speaker's political perspective, with the Government favouring the second but many other commentators the first.[2]

The British experience

The introduction of the purchaser–provider split has stimulated many exercises in explicit priority setting in the UK.[3] Each has included, to varying degrees, the views of health professionals, the public, and research based evidence. In contrast to most other countries, however, the British experience is characterised by the extent to which these attempts have been undertaken locally, by health authorities. Elsewhere such exercises have been conducted nationally[4-6] or, in the USA, at state level.[7] Indeed, the reluctance of the Government to become engaged in a national debate on priority setting and, in particular, the ethical issues that underpin it, has been striking.

A speech by the former Secretary of State for Health that set out the Government's views on this issue was noteworthy for the absence of any attempt to provide ethical principles to guide these many decision makers, or even to recognise that such principles might be needed.[8] Furthermore, the Health of the Nation strategy, which sets out the Government's priorities for health, as opposed to health services, ignored several ethical issues such as the widely held view that socioeconomic differentials in health should be addressed. This refusal to become involved in a national debate has been maintained despite many calls to do so.

This approach is consistent with Government policy throughout the public sector, which argues that those at local level are provided with resources to achieve their objectives and they must then choose how best to do so. The advocates of this policy see it as a means of empowering those with most knowledge of local circumstances. Its critics complain that the resources are inadequate to respond to the increasing amount of central, and often very detailed, direction and the consequences of changes in other Government policies.

An alternative approach

A recent report from Sweden offers an alternative approach.[9] The Swedish health service has many similarities with that in the UK. Some counties have introduced a purchaser–provider split, and since 1994 Sweden has spent about the same percentage of its gross domestic product on health. It too has had a series of local priority setting initiatives.[10] The new report provides a comprehensive agreed national statement on priorities.

The Swedish Priorities Commission was established by the Government to consider the responsibilities, demarcation, and role of healthcare services in the welfare state, to highlight the fundamental ethical principles that can furnish guidance and form a basis for open discussions, and recommend guidelines for priority setting in health services. The Commission comprised representatives of the five leading political parties, with none in a majority, and of central and local government. It worked in two stages. The first, from June 1992 to November 1993, involved administering questionnaires and consulting experts and other authorities. It also drew on examples of priority setting in other countries. The second phase began with the publication of a discussion document, which was circulated widely in November 1993[11] and was followed by a series of regional meetings, attitude surveys, and responses from interested parties.

Attitude surveys

There were four attitude surveys directed at each of the key interest groups. They included a nationwide random survey of 1500 people aged 18–84 years, which achieved a 78% response rate. This asked about the relative value to be placed on different forms of care and care for different age groups. A second questionnaire was designed to examine the attitudes of health professionals and was sent to 300 doctors and nurses. A third examined ethical values and concepts of justice among a sample of 168 politicians, 144 administrators, and 259 doctors. Finally, a study of the impact of changes in health service management was sent to 671 doctors and nurses in Stockholm. Subsequently the information collected and the views expressed on it were used to assemble a final report.[9]

Ethical frameworks

The report describes several examples of attempts to set priorities at national or state level such as those in Oregon, Norway, New Zealand, and the Netherlands. It finds each wanting in important aspects, usually their superficial exploration of ethical issues or their tendency to gloss over methodological problems in measuring efficiency. Specification of the ethical context is seen as crucial as there are many possible ethical frameworks within which it is possible to set priorities. A full discussion is beyond the scope of this article, but they include, for example: desert, in which judgments are made about who deserves what depending on their contribution to society or the extent to which they are seen as responsible for their illness; utilitarianism, or the greatest good for the greatest number; and need, in which individuals are offered treatment on the basis of their ability to benefit, however defined.

On the basis of the consultation process described above, the Commission established three ethical principles to underpin its work. These were, in order of importance: human dignity, need and solidarity, and cost efficiency. The human dignity principle is that all people have equal dignity and the same rights regardless of their personal characteristics and their function in the community, thus explicitly rejecting theories based on desert. The need and solidarity principle encompasses both the requirement to direct resources to those whose needs are greatest but also to pay special attention to those who are less able to voice their needs or exercise their rights. The cost efficiency principle is that there should be a "reasonable relation" between cost and effect, but it also notes that comparisons of interventions are possible only for the same diseases, thus rejecting some of the more ambitious utilitarian approaches such as those based on QALYs (quality adjusted life years). They also rejected or subordinated several other principles including ability to benefit, lottery, demand, and autonomy.

Priority groups

Arising from these principles, the report identifies client groups who should be accorded priority. Such priority is based largely on the seriousness of their illnesses. Although there was a widely held view among the public that, other things being equal, resources should go to the young rather than the old, the Commission rejected any link with chronological age but accepted that the consequences of the ageing process may be relevant. They also rejected some forms of prioritisation, such as those based on factors related to premature underweight babies, on whether injuries were self inflicted, on economic capacity, and on social position, and they argued that long term care should be protected from spending cuts.

These decisions thus imply, at least, an entitlement to medical assessment by those who suspect they may need care. The priority placed on them subsequently will depend on the nature of their condition. To facilitate discussion, nine categories of health care were generated (see box), as well as preventive interventions, considered separately.

Clinical and administrative priorities

The Commission explicitly recognised that the priorities of those responsible for planning and purchasing care may differ from those required to deliver it. It thus distinguished political or administrative prioritisation from clinical prioritisation. The first is population oriented, anonymous, and often planned in advance. The second is personal and often must reflect rapidly changing circumstances. This distinction led the Commission to generate a series of priorities (see box). In practice the two sets are almost the same, but in the case of clinical priorities life threatening illnesses have been separated from chronic diseases as they override all other priorities in terms of the need for speed of action.

Categories of health care

1 Care of life threatening diseases
2 Care of severe chronic diseases
3 Palliative terminal care
4 Care of persons with reduced autonomy
5 Habilitation/rehabilitation and provision of artificial aids
6 Care of minor acute and chronic diseases
7 Borderline cases
8 Care for reasons other than disease or injury
9 Care with no documented benefit
10 Prevention

Political or administrative priorities in Sweden

1 Treatment of life threatening acute diseases and diseases which, if left untreated, will lead to permanent disability or premature death. Treatment of severe chronic disease. Palliative terminal care. Care of people with reduced autonomy.
2 Prevention with a documented benefit. Habilitation/rehabilitation etc, as defined in the Health and Medical Services Act.
3 Treatment of less severe acute and chronic diseases.
4 Borderline cases.
5 Care for reasons other than disease or injury.

The Commission identified a series of borderline conditions where it questioned the justification for funding, arising from continuing uncertainty about what was appropriate. This uncertainty reflected widely differing views put before the Commission by various interest groups and included interventions for infertility (which it was felt were often, on balance, justified), and hormonal treatment for shortness of stature in the absence of an identifiable cause and psychotherapy where evidence of psychiatric illness is doubtful (both of which were felt to be rarely justified). Finally, it recommended that care for reasons other than disease or injury should not be communally funded.

Implementation

On implementation, the Commission explicitly avoids prescribing specific approaches such as guidelines or financial incentives. This derives from a consideration, informed by the surveys and other evidence, of the healthcare framework within which its recommendations will be set, including issues of ownership and the role of markets. Instead, it notes that successful implementation will depend on developing sufficient insight, determination, and ability at an administrative level and knowledge, leadership, and interest among clinicians. As noted in the title of the initial Swedish report, there are no easy solutions.[11] The Commission does, however, support the creation of advisory committees on prioritisation, with both lay and professional members, and has proposed a series of legislative changes to enshrine its proposed ethical basis in law.

Differences between Swedish and British approaches

The differences between the British and Swedish experiences are striking. The most obvious is that a document exists in Sweden whereas there is no equivalent in the UK. The Swedes have concentrated on tackling underlying principles, such as what general categories of ill health should receive greater priority and how priorities should be weighted. The Commission advocated that higher priorities should receive more resources than lower ones. It thus rejected other approaches such as only funding care for patients with priority 2 conditions once all priority 1 need has been met, or funding the first three priorities equally with nothing for categories four and five. This recognises the impossibility of developing and implementing detailed explicit and rigid guidelines[12]

In contrast, many British attempts have focused on methodological challenges such as the design of questionnaires and development of sampling frames to ascertain the views of the public.[13] Discussion of more fundamental issues, such as the relationship between the individual and the state and the ethical principles that should guide our thinking on it, have, with a few exceptions,[14] been almost completely lacking from the British debate.

What can we learn?

So what can Britain learn from the Swedes? They have clearly succeeded in stimulating a nationwide debate on priorities in health care, bringing together the views of all the key actors—the public, whose views were ascertained through surveys and public meetings; experts; health professionals; and political parties. The careful attention to detail has enabled them to identify the limitations of many of the technological fixes that have frequently been proposed, by, for example, saying explicitly that the benefits of health care "cannot possibly be stated in economic terms". This is consistent with both the theoretical arguments against expecting cost utility analysis to provide easy solutions[15] and the observation by Klein in evidence to the House of Commons Health Committee that such measures are not being used in practice.[16] This approach has also enabled them to tackle difficult issues such as how health care should be financed and organised and whether providers should be private or public. Of course, it is still too early to judge the success of their project, which will depend on the ability to implement it. At least it has provided a clear framework within which to move forward.

The next steps involve collating the responses from the many organisations to which the report has been distributed. Their comments were due by mid-October 1995, following which a draft bill was to be presented to Parliament in early 1996. The Commission's report is, however, already having an impact on debate about health care at local and national levels.

Question for Britain

The questions for Britain are twofold. The first is whether this approach could be adopted here. The second is that, if it cannot be, why not? In answer to the first question, there are many voices calling for national ethical guidance in the UK. The Commons Health Committee has called for "an honest and realistic set of explicit, well understood, ethical principles at national level to guide the NHS into the next century", suggesting that such principles should build on those implied by various Government documents: equity, public choice, and effective use of health service resources.[16] Interestingly, these are similar to those adopted by the Swedish commission. Unfortunately the Commons committee did not indicate how such principles might be arrived at, except to imply that they might be produced by the Government.

Clinical priorities in Sweden

1A Treatment of life threatening acute diseases. Treatment of diseases which, if left untreated, will lead to permanent disability or premature death.

1B Treatment of severe chronic diseases. Palliative terminal care. Care of people with reduced autonomy.

2 Individualised prevention during contacts with medical services. Habilitation/rehabilitation etc as defined in the Health and Medical Services Act.

3 Treatment of less severe acute and chronic diseases.

4 Borderline cases.

5 Care for reasons other than disease or injury.

The British Medical Association has sought to stimulate debate through a national conference and subsequent publication of the proceedings.[17] The need for a national view has also been expressed by the Royal College of Physicians, which has advocated the establishment of a National Council on Health Care Priorities,[18] although it gave more weight than the Swedes to expert rather than lay membership and to professional and technical rather than ethical issues. And any fears that national ethical guidance would conflict with local decision making, do not seem to be borne out by the calls for guidance made by many officers of health authorities.[16]

Despite these calls for national guidance, the Government has consistently rejected the idea of an authoritative national commission, thus effectively blocking it. So if this is not possible in the UK, why not?

Need for consensus

Perhaps the key issue, addressed explicitly by the Swedes, is the need for consensus. It is necessary, although not sufficient, that an ethical framework within which hard decisions will be made should command broad political support. Could this be achieved in the UK? In the current political context in the UK it is difficult to see how cross party agreement might emerge on anything as potentially contentious as this, given the divisions on most areas of social policy. Indeed, as noted above, it is not even possible to agree on whether to call this process rationing or priority setting.

The Swedish example would require a committee that includes all the main political parties as well as representatives of local government, with no party having a majority, something quite different from a parliamentary committee. Recent experience of cross party committees tackling difficult issues, such as members' financial interests, does not give cause for hope. In the more consensual politics before 1979 such an issue might have been tackled by a Royal Commission. These bodies lost favour with the Government in the 1980s,[19] although the Labour Party had stated that it would convene one to look at the related topic of long term care.[20] Even so, an appointed body composed of "the great and the good" does not have the democratic mandate necessary to yield legitimacy. Despite these difficulties, however, it is striking that the Swedish commission was working during a period, for Sweden, of unprecedented political polarisation and conflict, although this was still much less than in the UK in recent years.

Priority setting is an ethical issue

So a national priority setting commission seems unlikely to be established in the UK in the foreseeable future. This presents a major problem. If the adversarial and highly polarised nature of British politics makes it so difficult for politicians to offer guidance in priority setting, is it really fair of them to require health authorities and fundholders, both with even less democratic accountability, to do it for them? Moreover, while recognising the need to reflect local circumstances, it is far from clear that the emerging diversity in entitlement to treatment both between fundholders and health authorities and between different health authorities[16] is consistent with the views of the public.

It may not be possible to produce an ethical framework to underpin priority setting that reflects all the major ideological strands in British politics. But if this is indeed so then this must be explicitly recognised. We can then begin to address the reasons why. For now, the Swedish experience provides a reminder that setting priorities is fundamentally an ethical issue, requiring those involved at least to acquaint themselves with the differing theories of social justice and indicate where they stand in relation to them.

Acknowledgments

We thank Ingrid Petersson from the Swedish Ministry of Health and Social Affairs for helpful comments.

1 Abel-Smith B, Mossialos E, Figueras J, McKee M, Holland W. *Choices in health policy: an agenda for the European Union.* Aldershot: Dartmouth Press, 1995.
2 Smith R. Introduction In: Smith R, ed. *Rationing in action.* London: BMJ Publishing, 1993:vii-x.
3 Ham C. Priority setting in the NHS: Reports from six districts. In: Smith R, ed. *Rationing in action.* London: BMJ Publishing, 1993:59-71.
4 The Royal Ministry of Health and Social Welfare, Norway. *Retningslinjer for prioritering innen Norsk helesetjeneste.* Oslo: NOU, 1987:23.
5 *Choices in health care: A report by the Government Committee on Choices in Health Care.* Rijswijk, the Netherlands: Ministry of Health, Welfare and Cultural Affairs, 1992 (AJ Dunning, chairman).
6 National Advisory Committee. *Core services 1993/4.* Wellington: NAC, 1992.
7 Klein R. On the Oregon trail: rationing health care. BMJ 1991;**302**:1-2.
8 Bottomley V. Priority setting in the NHS. In: Smith R, ed. *Rationing in action.* London: BMJ Publishing, 1993:25-32.
9 Swedish Parliamentary Priorities Commission. *Priorities in health care: Ethics, economy, implementation.* Stockholm: Ministry of Health and Social Affairs, 1995:5.
10 Honigsbaum F, Calltorp J, Ham C, Holmstrvm S. *Priority setting processes for healthcare.* Oxford: Radcliffe, 1995.
11 Ministry of Health and Social Affairs. Health Care and Medical Priorities Commission. *No easy choices—the difficult priorities of health care.* Stockholm: Ministry of Health and Social Affairs, 1993:93.
12 McKee M, Clarke A. Guidelines, enthusiasms, uncertainty, and the limits to purchasing. BMJ 1995;**310**:101-4.
13 Bowling A, Jacobson B, Southgate L. Health service priorities: explorations in consultation of the public and health professionals on priority setting in an inner London health district. *Soc Sci Med* 1993;**37**:851-7
14 Chadwick R. Justice in priority setting. In: Smith R, ed. *Rationing in action.* London: BMJ Publishing, 1993:85-95.

15 Carr-Hill R. Allocating resources to health care: is the QALY (quality adjusted life year) a technical solution to a political problem? *Int J Health Serv* 1991:21:351-63.
16 House of Commons Health Committee. *Priority setting in the NHS: Purchasing. First Report Session 1994-95.* London: HMSO, 1995 (HC 134-I).
17 Smith R, ed. *Rationing in action.* London: BMJ Publishing, 1993.
18 Royal College of Physicians. Setting priorities in the NHS: a framework for decision making. *J Coll Physicians Lond* 1995;29:379-80.
19 Jenkins S. *Accountable to none: the Tory nationalisation of Britain.* Harmondsworth: Hamish Hamilton, 1995.
20 Labour Party. *Renewing the NHS. Labour's agenda for a healthier Britain.* London: The Labour Party, 1995.

14 Setting priorities: is there a role for citizens' juries?

JO LENAGHAN, BILL NEW, ELIZABETH MITCHELL

One sixth of health authorities are now explicitly excluding certain treatments from public provision.[1] Who is making these decisions, and according to what criteria? What opportunities do the public have to challenge or be involved in these decisions? As Anne Bowling has pointed out, obtaining a representative view from the public can be difficult, and the methodology of ranking lists of treatments and services can be criticised as superficial in relation to the complexity of the decision to be made.[2] The Institute for Public Policy Research in partnership with Cambridge and Huntingdon Health Authority has recently piloted the first citizens' jury in the UK in an attempt to develop a more sophisticated technique for involving the public in these difficult decisions.[3]

Methods

Professional recruiters (Opinion Leader Research) were given a demographic breakdown of the Cambridge and Huntingdon area, and 16 people were selected by stratified random sampling to represent their community. The jury sat for four days, and during this time the members were presented with information to help them to reach a number of decisions. Jurors were asked to consider how priorities for purchasing health care should be set, according to what criteria, and what role, if any, the public should have in these decisions. Expert witnesses gave evidence, and jurors were given the opportunity to question them before debating the issues among themselves. All of their discussions were recorded, and jurors were asked to fill in questionnaires before and after the event on issues of health policy, both as individuals and as a group, so that we could obtain some quantitative and qualitative data.

212

Results

The citizens' jury heard evidence from Ron Zimmern, Director of Public Health at Cambridge and Huntingdon Health Authority, who explained how the health authority currently sets priorities. The jurors developed their own criteria for purchasing health care and debated whether quality was more important than quantity in the context of finite resources, after hearing evidence about single and dual chamber pacemakers in order to help them address the issues. A majority (12/16) felt that quantity was more important than quality in the context of a finite budget. The jurors were also asked to consider whether a health authority should give priority to effective treatments for minor problems or to treatments of unproved effectiveness for life threatening conditions. To help them decide about this issue, jurors heard evidence from doctors and patients about deviated nasal septa. Most jurors favoured giving greater priority to effective treatments for minor problems but were keen for health authorities to continue to fund treatments of unproved value in the interests of medical research and progress.

On the third day the jury considered whether priorities should be set at a local or a national level. Professor Maurice Lessof gave evidence on behalf of the Royal College of Physicians and outlined the case for creating a national council for priority setting.[4] Philip Hunt, Director of the National Association of Health Authorities and Trusts, argued that priority setting should be left to the local health authorities, and Frank Honigsbaum, a health economist, explained what strategies other countries used to deal with these issues. After much discussion and debate, at the end of the day all 16 jurors agreed that there should be a national council for priority setting. Thirteen of the jurors thought that the role of this body should be to set guidelines for decision making at the local level; two jurors thought that a national body should be proscriptive, defining what is and is not available on the NHS; and one juror felt that a national council for priority setting could do both. This finding was repeated in a questionnaire which each juror was given at the end of the fourth day to fill in privately.

Most of the jurors (15/16) thought that there should be an element of public involvement in developing guidelines for priority setting at a local and national level, although most thought that public opinion should only be taken into account along with other interests. Some jurors were keen to see lay representation on the national council for priority setting, but others thought that a body like a citizens' jury could scrutinise the work of this council and inform it of the public's opinion on specific issues. All of the jurors pointed out that if the public were to be involved in the decision making process then people would need a lot more information about the issues concerned. There was a strong feeling that the national council for priority setting should not be political—most jurors thought

213

that doctors, ethicists, health economists, lay people, and even health managers should sit on the council, but nobody voted for the involvement of politicians.

At the end of the citizens' jury, jurors were asked to reach a number of decisions, and their recommendations were written up in a report that was submitted to Cambridge and Huntingdon Health Authority for consideration. The commissioning authority is not bound by the decision as the aim is to enrich rather than replace the existing decision making process. However, the authority should take the findings of the jury seriously, and if it does not follow the recommendations of the jurors then it must set out its reasons for this.

Discussion of the process

This pilot jury was also concerned with evaluating issues of process: how did the jury cope with the questions; how were its deliberations managed; how much information should be provided; and how should jurors be recruited and reimbursed?

Choosing a question

The crucial issue is the choice of question that the jury is asked to address. In Huntingdon, the jury was given a broad set of questions concerning how decisions relating to priority setting in the NHS should be made. Initially the jurors found this difficult. It was hard for them to assimilate all the information necessary to address these issues, and they were not clear what, precisely, they were required to answer. One interesting aspect of the jurors' reaction was their initial nervousness about whether, in this context, they ought to be involved in making decisions on public policy. They asked why the elected or appointed bodies were not making these decisions and whether members of the public were competent, technically or otherwise, to do so in their place.

Over the course of the jury, the jurors gained in confidence, but clearly the more broad and open ended the question, the longer the jury will need to sit and the more difficulty it will find in suggesting concrete proposals. When the jurors were presented with a choice between a clear set of options, such as whether priorities should be set at local or national level, they found it easier to deliberate and reach a conclusion.

There are two models for citizens' juries: a "deliberative" model involving broad, open ended questions where the jury is engaged in a process of guiding policy makers and offering feedback and opinion from the local community; and a "decision making" model, where the jury adjudicates

214

on a "live" issue involving a clear set of options and where a statutory body has found it difficult to reach a decision using standard procedures. Both models could improve the democratic process; the second might also improve the legitimacy with which controversial decisions are made.

Jury deliberation

Another important issue was the organisation of the jury's deliberations. The central problem was one of group dynamics: how could the moderators ensure that all the members of the jury have adequate opportunity to express their opinions? Not surprisingly, some jurors were more articulate, confident and experienced, and better educated. They tended to dominate the discussions when all the jurors were present. To address this issue, the jury was split into two smaller groups, one of men and one of women. As a simple expedient, this worked well—those who were quieter in sessions involving the whole group gained confidence in a smaller group, although other methods of organising small group discussions need to be explored.

In managing the jury's deliberations, the role of the moderator is crucial. The moderator acts as a kind of chairperson, ensuring that discussions run on time, that all jurors have a chance to participate, and that witnesses keep to their brief and answer the questions that are put to them. Moderators also need to ensure that the discussion stays on the chosen topic, while at the same time allowing opportunities for jurors to suggest their own witnesses and questions. Clearly this is a skilled job: the approach in Huntingdon was to use moderators with no experience or knowledge of the subject matter; an alternative would be to use a neutral "expert". The problem with the first strategy is that witnesses may be able to manipulate the jury by using their specialist knowledge; with the second, the danger is that bias may creep into the proceedings.

Information

There is a question about how much background information to provide, and how to deal with "points of fact". Jurors felt they would have benefited from background briefings, both relating to the overall question at stake and the individual witnesses' presentations. There may be a case for supplying the jury with a briefing paper from a neutral expert before the jury convenes, and encouraging witnesses to supply a one page summary of their argument, also in advance. The difficulty is ensuring that this information is neutral.

Clarifying questions from jurors about points of fact is even more problematic. There could be an "expert" on hand to provide this information, but no individual is all knowledgeable, and having a single person undertaking the role might introduce bias. However, some procedure for dealing with factual inquiries is necessary.

Recruitment and reimbursement

The jurors were selected at random to represent the sociodemographic characteristics of their community. Although this did not present problems in Huntingdon, in other areas there may be a need to resolve difficulties for jurors for whom English is not their first language.

It was felt that significantly more than the 16 jurors who were recruited would have made the sessions hard to manage; however, more experience is needed of other jury sizes. To retain impartiality it may also be necessary to vet jurors to ensure that none has a vested interest: for example, should a clinician be allowed to take part in a jury discussing issues of priority setting when he or she might stand to benefit from a particular decision? Jurors were reimbursed with £250 for the four days. They seemed satisfied with this payment—no juror dropped out and attendance was almost 100% over the period the jury sat.

Conclusion

The Cambridge and Huntingdon citizens' jury has shown that, given enough time and information, the public is willing and able to contribute to the debate about priority setting in health care. We are hopeful that this method, in conjunction with the more traditional techniques, may offer us a meaningful way of involving the public in decisions about priority setting in health.[5] Decision makers at a local and national level should seize this opportunity to show that they are willing not only to listen to but to act on the voice of the public.

1 Redmayne S. *Reshaping the NHS: strategies and priorities and resource allocation*. Birmingham: National Association of Health Authorities and Trusts, 1995.
2 Bowling A. Health care rationing: The public's debate. *BMJ* 1996;**312**:670–4.
3 Coote A, Kendall L, Stewart J. *Citizens' juries*. London: Institute for Public Policy Research, 1994.
4 Royal College of Physicians. Setting priorities in the NHS: a framework for decision making. *J Coll Physicians Lond* 1995;**29**:379–80.
5 Cooper L, Coote A, Davies A, Jackson C. *Tackling the democratic deficit in health*. London: Institute for Public Policy Research, 1995.

15 The Asbury draft policy on ethical use of resources

ROGER CRISP, TONY HOPE, DAVID EBBS

Many doctors find themselves torn between two contradictory principles: to do the best for the individual patient and to be responsible for an overall budget that is insufficient for the best care for each individual patient. Little guidance is available for doctors on how to resolve this conflict. Crisp *et al* present a draft document that one fundholding general practice has developed to clarify the ethical basis for rationing decisions. We invited three interested professionals to comment on the draft.

- The primary aim of this policy document is to provide a principled basis for the distribution of financial and medical resources within the practice.
- The practice is assumed to have a responsibility to provide health care within budgetary constraints. It is also recognised that differences of opinion between partners about the use of resources are inevitable. A secondary aim of the document, therefore, is to provide machinery for making decisions in cases of disagreement.
- We believe that it is important to consult widely before producing the final document. This draft will therefore be discussed with other members of the practice, with patient forums, and with professionals and the public.
- The document is intended to be available to anyone who requests it.
- This document is the outcome of many meetings attended by the partners. Advice has been sought when appropriate from others outside the practice.
- The document is concerned with how the partnership should come to decisions about the distribution of the resources under its control. The resources available to the partnership are fewer than the partnership considers ideal. In producing these guidelines, the partnership does not wish to imply that it endorses as ideal the level of funding available to it.

Ethical background to allocation of scarce resources

In preparing this document, we considered in particular three general theories pertinent to the allocation of medical resources. Each theory

217

focuses on different values. We believe that decisions on the use of resources should not be based on only one value. Several values are at stake, and the judgment of the partners will be needed to balance these values in particular cases.

Three ethical theories

Quality adjusted life years (QALYs)—The theory of QALYs[1] was developed specifically to address the issue of how limited resources for health care should be distributed. It focuses on maximising the welfare of patients. Patient welfare, according to the QALY theory, is the product of length of life and the quality (to the particular person) of that life. Various empirical means have been suggested for measuring the "quality adjustment".

The fact that a certain treatment will produce greater patient welfare than another is a reason—though not necessarily an overriding reason—for that treatment to be chosen. It will thus be important that the partners have as much information as possible about the impact of various treatments on patient welfare.

Needs theory— Needs theory[2,3] is based on the view that some patients have a special claim on resources that rests not on the mere maximising of overall welfare but on their greater need for treatment. The most thoroughly worked out version of needs theory is that of John Rawls, who emphasises the value of fairness.

We believe that medical practice should not aim solely to maximise overall patient welfare, because it matters how this wellbeing is distributed among patients. Consider the following hypothetical case of hernia treatments versus kidney treatment. A doctor could treat either 100 otherwise healthy people for hernias or one very sick person for severe and debilitating kidney problems. On the assumption that each hernia treatment provides one unit of benefit and the kidney treatment provides 50 units, the total number of units of benefit for the kidney treatment is half that of the hernia treatments.

A principle according to which patient welfare should be maximised suggests that there is no reason to treat the person who is worse off—namely, the patient with kidney disease—because he or she is worse off. But another value, that of fairness, requires that some consideration be given to patients who are worse off, perhaps in terms of meeting basic needs, independently of how much patient welfare will be produced by treating them.

Lottery theory—The lottery theory[4] arises from the view that in many health care situations there is no good reason, when a choice exists, for treating person A rather then person B, or vice versa. In such situations the value of procedural fairness suggests giving both an equal chance of treatment.

Patient autonomy

So far the values of patient welfare and substantive and procedural fairness have been mentioned. A fourth value is the autonomy of patients. We believe that allowing patients as much say as is practically possible in their treatment is a good thing in itself.

Imagine that two treatments are available for a certain condition, each of which has different side effects. One treatment is slightly more expensive than the other. Allowing patients to choose their treatment will respect their autonomy. There are limits to autonomy, however, because of the partners' responsibility to provide health care within a specific budget. Thus if two treatments differed greatly in price patient choice may not be possible.

Plurality of values

We believe that a plurality of values does not rule out rational decision making—in fact, such decision making requires that all these values be taken into account. In some cases—for example, when a great gain can be achieved in patient welfare by treating those patients who are not in fact the worst off—it may be rational to decide to produce this gain. But in some cases it may be worth sacrificing overall gain to offer some priority to those worse off.

Process of decision making

In the absence of a single overriding theory or an ethical principle that provides for all circumstances, we believe that it is critically important to establish a methodical process for making decisions.

Partners' monthly and policy meetings

As the decisions depend on the particular facts of each case, as much clinical and financial information as possible must be available. The decisions will be made at the monthly practice meetings. The values underlying these decisions are those discussed above, and this section of the document provides a constitutional framework for discussion.

We believe that it is important to be open about rationing policy. This document serves as a statement of policy. The partners' monthly meetings will be an important forum in which this policy statement will be interpreted in specific instances. If there is any major conflict between partners in interpreting this policy statement or if a change in policy is proposed then a specific policy meeting will be called.

Patient information admissible to discussion

In the discussions about allocation of resources any information about a patient and his or her situation is considered admissible. Both positive and negative bias from the patient's advocate—for example, the partner most involved in that patient's care—may distort the presentation of the case. We believe, however, that the patient is protected from such bias by the presence of the other members of the group. It is for this reason that both policy statements and decisions about choices between individual patients (necessary because of rationing) must be made by the group and not by individuals. We considered whether we should regard some information about patients—such as whether, they have a learning disability—as inadmissible to the discussion. We concluded that if some information were inadmissible this may wrongly affect a partner's judgment without it being clear that the partner's judgment was affected. We therefore decided to allow all patient information to be discussed, but the partners must ensure that the decisions made are informed by this policy document.

Final decisions

As the partners carry legal responsibility for the use of the resources, they have to make the final decisions about what should become policy. The partners should, however, consult as widely as appropriate in drawing up this policy statement, in interpreting it, and in developing it. Some other members of the practice would probably also be present at most policy meetings. We foresee a time when the composition of the policy group—that is, the group that makes the final decisions about rationing policy—will be multiprofessional and representative of a wide range of different views. We are looking at a model for this process of wider consultation, so that the views of the team are incorporated in the policy.

Annual report

In addition to preparing and developing this policy document, the partnership undertakes to provide an annual report. This report will summarise the issues raised—at both the partners' monthly meetings and policy meetings—and the ensuing discussion when these concern issues of resource allocation. The annual report will be made public along with the most recent policy statement. It is important, therefore, that both the policy statement and the annual report do not breach any individual patient's confidentiality.

Values held by the partnership: general policy

The central ethical principle that guides the practice of medicine in this partnership is that of "the best interests of each patient". The partnership will try to provide whatever medical care is in the best interests of each individual patient.

This policy statement has been drawn up, however, because the limitation on funding means that the partnership may not always be able to pursue the best interests of every patient in every circumstance. As our practice is fundholding, a considerable portion of the total medical budget is under our direct control. We therefore wish to clarify for ourselves, our employees, and our patients what principles and working practices should guide us when budgetary constraints prevent us from being able to pursue the best interests of every patient. However, for most patients, most of the time, we envisage that we will be able to provide the care that is in each patient's best interests.

When the best interests of every patient cannot be met, a decision about what should be done will normally be made by the partners after discussion at a specifically convened meeting (the partners' monthly meeting). This meeting will normally be cancelled only when a patient's situation is one for which an agreed policy already exists.

All the values identified by the various ethical theories will be considered before a decision is reached. Partners have different views on the way in which these values are balanced. The mechanism for making a decision will be through consensus, and if necessary through voting, at the partnership meeting. We believe that this mechanism is preferable to individual partners making decisions for two reasons: it ensures clarification and identification of various points of view, and it ensures that individual partners' responses to specific patients do not, illegitimately, affect the choices made.

Values held by the partnership: specific issues

Age of patients

We do not wish to deny treatment on the basis of age—that is, the partnership rejects any policy that states that no one over a particular age

221

should *ipso facto* not be allowed a specific treatment. Hospitals, however, which are not controlled by the partnership, may operate such a policy for some treatments, and the partnership may be unable to find suitable alternative treatment. But the partnership will do what it can to ensure treatment and will not itself deny treatment on the basis of age.

Situations may occur rarely in which the partnership has to choose which of two patients should have priority in receiving some beneficial and expensive treatment. In such cases a decision about how to proceed will be made at the partnership meeting. It will be legitimate to consider any factor as at least potentially relevant to making a decision. This does not imply that any factor that can be considered will be thought relevant in a specific case. For example, the patients' ages may be considered and found relevant. This is because the partnership believes that two ethical values may be relevant: (1) how long each patient is likely to live to enjoy the benefit of the treatment (a value endorsed by the QALY perspective), and (2) "the fair innings argument", which highlights a value in justice which the partners consider to have some weight. The fair innings argument suggests that to "treat the older person, letting the younger person die, would thus be inherently inequitable in terms of years of life lived: the younger person would get no more years than the relatively few he has already had, whereas the older person . . . will get several years more".[5]

Chronic problems affecting welfare

With regard to patients with chronic problems affecting welfare—for example, learning disabilities or chronic physical ill health—the partnership does not endorse the values embedded in the QALY theory. A person's learning disability or rheumatoid arthritis, for example, is not a reason for either lowering or increasing his or her priority over people without those problems, although what is in the best interests of the patient may be affected by his or her chronic problems.

Patients' responsibility for conditions

The partnership rejects any general policy that denies specific treatment to a patient on the grounds that he or she has brought the condition on himself or herself. The partnership believes that if the patient would benefit from medical treatment then it should be available, regardless of the cause of the condition. However, if the partnership has to choose which of two patients should have priority in receiving some beneficial and expensive treatment then the issue of a patient's responsibility for having induced the problem might be considered relevant.

Dependants

In drawing up this policy document, the partnership considered the following fictional situation to help it to clarify its views. Two patients need the same treatment for the same life threatening condition. Patient A is a brilliant surgeon who saves hundreds of lives a year; she is a single parent with three young children. Patient B is unemployed and has no dependants. Resources are available for treating only one patient.

Should the issue of dependants ever affect in any way the priority of patients for access to scarce resources? In the fictional case above, do the facts that patient A through her work has a beneficial effect on many other people and that she has dependent children provide a reason for giving her a higher priority?

The partners believe that patient A's work is not relevant to decisions on priority; they do not think that they should be making any judgments about the value of patients to society in deciding issues of resource allocation.

However, the partners believe that if, as in this case, a patient has dependent children then this could be a factor in increasing the priority for scarce resources if those resources will affect the patient's ability to care for the dependent children.

Paying for treatment

- All patients have the right to seek private treatment either by referral from the partnership or independently of it.
- Patients have a right to NHS treatment as laid down in various statutes.
- Some treatments—for example, paracetamol syrup for children—are advised to a large number of patients. Under the terms of service with the NHS, patients have the right to an NHS prescription for these treatments. Prescriptions for these treatments, because they are common, are a high expense to the practice's drug budget; the money could be spent on other treatment. The cost of a prescription for any one patient, however, is low. The partners believe that, despite a patient's right to obtain a prescription, it is right to inform most patients (or their parents) that they could buy such drugs themselves, although if the drug would not be purchased then a prescription, when clinically indicated, should be given.

Relation to District Health Authority

The practice will normally expect to follow any District Health Authority guidelines for funding specific procedures. The partners accept that, at this

223

Factors in deciding priority for allocation of scarce resources

May be relevant
Age
Dependency on the patient of people who are close relatives
The patient's responsibility for causing his or her condition

Not relevant
Value of a patient to society
Value of a patient's life to that patient
Race
Sex
Dependency on the patient of people who are not close relatives

---

stage, most authority decisions have been made on the basis of good reasons after appropriate consideration of the available evidence. The partners will, however, ask the District Health Authority for the reasons behind its policy. A distinction exists between purely clinical and ethical reasons for refusing to fund treatments. The partners believe that it could be appropriate to act contrary to the authority's guidelines if they found the reasons behind the policy inadequate. They envisage that this is more likely to be the case with regard to ethical guidelines than with clinical guidelines. If the reason behind an authority guideline is found to be inadequate the practice policy would be determined after discussion at a partnership meeting.

The partners believe that it would be undesirable to create a local two tier service, and this should be avoided whenever possible. To help to prevent a two tier service the partners should be aware of monetary constraints forced on local non-fundholding practices by the district health authority. The partners should adopt policies at variance with those of non-fundholding practices only after careful consideration.

At present no funding will be available from the general practice budget for alternative therapies such as homoeopathy and osteopathy.

Budgeting

The partners do not believe that they should directly profit financially from money intended for patient care.

Buildings, expansion, improvement, new projects

As with the cost–rent scheme, in which we have an interest, we believe that appropriate resources should be allocated in a regional strategy for programmes in which appreciable expansion in establishment is needed to take account of changing demography and population growth. It is the responsibility of the Family Health Services Authority and District Health Authority to take appropriate action to provide adequate premises for accommodating general medical services. Money intended for patient care should not be used for this purpose.

Future budgets may contain development money that could be used for building costs. Such necessary work should be modest and functional. If the fundholding budget is underspent, and all agreed quality standards relating to clinical care have been achieved, the practice should discuss how best to spend the money, focusing on improvement in patient care.

Equipment

Before the practice became fundholding all equipment costs were the legitimate expense of the practice, but now planned savings can be used to buy items for patient care. We believe that the practice should be well equipped and that when a piece of equipment will directly benefit patient care in offering new services, improving existing services, or in saving expenditure elsewhere—for example, by buying an audiometer or tympanometer—it is justifiable to spend fundholding money.

End of life

The QALY theory is likely to result in few resources being put into terminal care. This is because, however much such care might enhance the quality of the patient's life, there will not be much quantity of life. Terminal care is therefore likely to be expensive when measured in terms of the cost per QALY.

We believe that good care at the end of life is an important aspect of medical care and that the quality of life then and the manner in which a person dies have an importance that is not captured by the idea of welfare in terms of life years. This is true because of the importance of how a person's life ends both to that person and to the person's close relatives. Good terminal care therefore might be considered to be a need.

Informing patients

We believe that patients should be told which policies—relevant to the allocation of resources—the partnership is following. Such policies include not only those specified in this document but also clinical protocols that have been developed at least in part as a response to budgetary constraints. The partnership might develop, for example, a protocol for treating a particular condition that states that treatment A is normally to be preferred in the first instance to treatment B. This protocol might be developed because, although treatment B is slightly better—for example, it may have fewer unwanted side effects—it is much more expensive. Any such protocol developed by the partners will be made public and will be available to patients in the same way as this policy statement.

Standards of clinical care: partners' responsibilities, to whom and for what

Our responsibilities are to individual patients—to provide high quality care. High quality care is care that is appropriate to the patient's needs and expectations based on logical rationale and validated by accepted scientific evidence. It should not be determined by availability or cost when a choice of treatment is being made.

We have an obligation to provide the highest quality of care at the best value for money, which means that we should follow agreed guidelines, procedures, and protocols of care and be aware of the costs of various equivalent options.

We have a responsibility to the patient to choose the most effective treatment that also represents the best value. We also have responsibility to assess the health needs of our local populations and to represent these to those authorities that deal with locality funding.

To fulfil these responsibilities we should:

- Collect and consider all existing agreed district protocols and guidelines and follow those that have been scientifically validated
- Review contract negotiations with providers to avoid waste of resources by unnecessary repetition of investigations, outpatient appointments, and follow ups (reports and regular review should be made of these and appropriate purchaser–provider locality meetings set up)
- Validate in house protocols by research and regularly audit agreement of and adherence to these protocols
- Make representation to supplement funds when the budget or resources are inadequate to fund high quality care based on acceptable criteria; when funds are not forthcoming, we should share our concerns with our patients, the public, and any influential public figures
- Agree policy decisions relating to standards of care with all relevant professionals and make these public for scrutiny.

1 Bell JM, Mendus S. *Philosophy and medical welfare*. Cambridge: Cambridge University Press, 1988.

2 Rawls J. *A theory of justice*. Cambridge, MA: Harvard University Press, 1971.
3 Daniels N. *Just health care*. Cambridge: Cambridge University Press, 1985.
4 Harris J. *The value of life*. London: Routledge, 1985.
5 Lockwood M. Quality of life and resource allocation. In: Bell JM, Mendus S, eds. *Philosophy and medical welfare*. Cambridge: Cambridge University Press, 1988:33–55.

Commentary: Guidelines for rationing resemble process of family decision making

DAVID C THOMASMA

The origin of the verb "to ration" comes from the Latin *ratio*, reason. Rationing, or providing guidelines for the use of resources, is a profoundly human activity, arising from our capacity to reason, especially our capacity to reason with an eye to the future and plan accordingly. As rationing is a human act, it participates in the moral character of all such acts. Therefore the effort to ration resources can be unjust, morally neutral, or a virtue, depending on the motives of those rationing, the qualities of the item to be rationed, and the goals and purposes of providing a plan for allocating resources. In all three instances, rationing arouses the most complex concerns about being fair to others with whom we live in community.

I take unjust rationing to be any form of either allocating or denying resources on indefensible bases—either inadequate versions of justice, equity, and fairness (such as discriminating on the basis of race, creed, religion, sex, age) or a hidden or covert basis that may in itself be adequate and fair but has not been adopted openly by the population that is affected by such a basis. The Asbury draft document addresses both of these concerns by making public a proposed basis for decision making in challenging circumstances. Furthermore, the proposal itself entails public discussion when providing resources or withholding them would challenge the partners' ultimate value of addressing the needs of individual patients in the context of the whole practice. The practice partnership's ultimate value is based on medical need and yet, as foreseen, will be circumscribed in individual cases by the common good of all those covered.

Morally neutral rationing would occur when people affected would not deserve the items to be rationed or allocated—for example, gifts of sweets for all the patients who come before 10 am. Those who arrive after that time are not discriminated against by the cut off, because the item rationed is a gift and not due to them by the practice. The contract about coverage may limit the partners' obligations to provide a treatment that is expensive and of little proved or even contested benefit—for example, bone marrow transplantation for advanced breast cancer. Not providing this treatment, then, would be morally neutral because it was explicitly ruled out by the contract and not due to the patients covered by it.

Morally good rationing occurs when allocation is based on public criteria, in fairness to all covered patients, with a goal of improving the welfare of all by enhancing the wellbeing of each individual as far as possible. None the less, the patients covered in a practice have a right to appeal against decisions that are made for the common good, as the partners' public meetings would do.

As the oldest of seven children, I was struck by how much the practice guidelines for allocation resemble a process of family decision making, albeit far more complex. Public discussion of difficult cases that fall outside the norm resemble family discussions of new needs that arise that fall outside a real or even anticipated budget—a son's need for spectacles, or a daughter's opportunity for cello lessons. A family's decision to forgo opportunities owing to budgetary constraints does not itself demean or diminish the personhood of the children. In a large family, as one of my nephews put it, "you don't always get what you want—you take what you are given".

So despite the alienation and depersonalisation that characterise the late twentieth century, the difficulties that modern medicine faces in providing a just form of medical care lead to the formulation of a new and improved concept of community. We are forced by scarcity of resources and by the commitment to act in the best interests of patients to create a more formal and explicit ideal of a community of healing, similar to that described by Crisp *et al* in the Asbury draft. They are to be commended for their commitment to carrying out the hard decisions.

Commentary: Courageous attempt, but needs clarification

PETER DORMER

The Asbury draft policy is a courageous and decent attempt at clarifying the ways that difficult moral decisions on treatment could be taken in general practice. The document is muddled, however, and Crisp *et al* swing between moral high handedness and hand wringing uncertainty.

I do not believe that Crisp *et al* have sorted out what they mean when (1) they argue that they want to allow patients as much say as possible in their treatment and (2) they say that they believe a plurality of values is necessary in making rational decisions. They give an example of a patient being offered two treatments, each with different side effects, with one treatment costing slightly more than the other. The patient can choose. Big deal. It is not a moral problem. Yet they then say that if the two treatments differ widely in price then the patient may not be allowed a choice. That is where the real issue lies. Will the patient be told or consulted about the fact that he or she cannot have treatment A because it is too expensive? And what about the patient who is refused treatment A for this reason but who could more easily tolerate the side effects of treatment A than those of the cheaper treatment B?

Crisp *et al* say that they are pluralists. They are not. They rule out five values as irrelevant to their decision making process. The values that they reject include "the value of a patient to society" and "the value of a patient's life to that patient".

I think that the authors are right to rule out a patient's value to society (partly because I am not sure that I would welcome an audit on my own value). None the less, if they had to choose between a saint and a rotter, each of equal age and each without dependants, then how would they solve the crisis? Their document does not tell us. Would Crisp *et al* explain their dilemma to the two patients? If they did would they haul the rotter in and appeal to him or her to do the decent thing just for once? Would they gaze hopefully at the saint, counting on the likelihood that he or she would jump at the chance of self sacrifice? Or would they inform neither patient about the moral difficulty and spin a coin? In the circumstances this might be an ethically justifiable act.

Ruling out the value of a patient's life to that patient seems to undermine "a patient's best interests". How would Crisp *et al* make a judgment on a person's best interests if they do not take into account the value of a patient's life to that patient? As a patient myself, I have found that one of several things that has made the care I receive feel moral, kind, and efficient is that each doctor and nurse seems interested enough in how I value my life for this to be a factor in my treatment.

Crisp *et al* should continue to explain their criteria, but they should stay clear of philosophy because it is not doing the job they want it to do: it is not supporting or clarifying their principles. This document is not yet ready for distribution to patients—it would confuse them. Moreover, the authors should know that they can afford to be blunt and tell patients, "You cannot always have what you want". Many patients do understand.

Commentary: Commendable but confused

PETER TOON

In resource allocation, as in the courts, it is necessary not only that justice be done but also that it be seen to be done. The obscurity of how, why, and by whom rationing decisions are made in the NHS contrasts sadly with the openness of British courts.

The purchaser–provider split made it possible for there to be greater clarity about how healthcare resources are allocated. It is surprising therefore that, despite widespread criticism of the ethical propriety of fundholding, fundholders have rarely published the principles that guide their actions. The Asbury practice's decision to do so is therefore to be welcomed.

Macintyre argues that the reason we find moral problems so intractable is that we live in a fragmented moral universe, with no coherent tradition of agreed moral axioms.[1] He suggested in despair that, in such a situation, the only solution for doctors is to advertise their ethical principles alongside their consulting hours.[2] Although he was thinking of doctors as providers rather than purchasers, this document moves towards adopting this suggestion.

An interesting result of setting down the decision making processes so clearly is the demonstration of the extent to which the general practitioner is given the role of "philosopher king"[3] in the primary care led NHS. Crisp et al justify their procedures on the basis of their legal accountability, but perhaps procedures incorporating more representation of other healthcare workers and of the practice population might be not only more democratic but also more comfortable for those who are ultimately legally accountable.

The commitment that the partners should not profit from savings invested in buildings is reassuring. This is a point on which the accountability framework is still far from satisfactory.[4] The document would be strengthened, however, if legal mechanisms to avoid such improper use—for example, charitable trusts—were specified.

Overall, however, the document's sharpness as a moral tool is questionable. The key to its weakness is found in the section discussing plurality of values and in the last paragraph in the section on general policy considering values. These indicate either that the partners cannot articulate their fundamental moral values (not uncommon, even among intelligent and well educated people) or, more likely, that they are working in different parts of Macintyre's fragmented moral universe. Certainly the three theories of just allocation that they mention are incommensurable in exactly the

230

way Macintyre discusses. The result is that many sections that commendably address important issues—such as age and self inflicted illness—include provisos that suggest that in the end decisions will be fudged.

However, the only way for a group to reach clarity over such difficult issues may be to start with such an ambiguous document and apply it to hard cases, which will either refine the tool or break it. It will therefore be interesting to see the results of the first year of its use. One might hope to see the partnership draw towards a better consensus as they use their framework to develop a moral tradition. Not all ethicists are as pessimistic as Macintyre in believing that these difficulties cannot be reconciled in an intellectually coherent way.[5]

1 Macintyre A. *After virtue—a study in moral theory*, 2nd edn. London: Duckworth, 1985.
2 MacIntyre A. Patients as agents. In: Spicker SF, Engelhart HT, eds. *Philosophical medical ethics, its nature and significance*. Dortrecht/Boston: Reidel, 1977.
3 Plato. *The republic*. London: Dent, 1992.
4 NHS Executive. *An accountability framework for GP fundholding—towards a primary care led NHS*. Heywood: NHSE Health Publications Unit, 1995.
5 Doyal L, Gough I. *A theory of human need*. London: Macmillan Education, 1991.

16 A purchaser experience of managing new expensive drugs: interferon-β

E ROUS, A COPPEL, J HAWORTH, S NOYCE

Interferon-β represents a drug company's dream ticket—the first new product for a chronic incurable disease that is relatively common and has a variable course. This drug is one of the first of the new biotechnological treatments for multiple sclerosis, all of which are likely to be relatively expensive drugs. This chapter describes the preparations undertaken by purchasing authorities in the North West region before the licensing of interferon-β. To our knowledge this is the first time such a major coordinated effort has been made by NHS purchasers to pre-empt the consequences of one drug.

Conclusions of published trial of drug

One published trial of interferon-β showed that it reduced the exacerbation rate in patients with relapsing–remitting disease.[1] The study population was aged 18–50 years and without important disability. The two year data demonstrated exacerbation rates of 1·27 per patient per year in the placebo group, 1·17 in the first treatment group (1·6 MIU dose), and 0·84 in the second treatment group (8 MIU). The difference between the placebo group and the second treatment group was significant: $p = 0·0001$. Technically, the trial demonstrated clinical effectiveness but not an effect on disability, which is the outcome that matters to purchasers and patients.

Purchasers need to be able to answer several questions when making a judgment about this drug:

- Is the reported reduction in exacerbation rate clinically important?
- Is there a subgroup of patients who would gain greater benefit from the drug?

Table 16.1   Comparative costs for three drugs

Drug	Cost per hospital inpatient day prevented (£)	Estimated annual cost in North West Region (£m)
Interferon-β	23 584	30
Clozapine[2,3]	33	9.9
Dornase α[4,5]	2857	6.1

- If the results are clinically important how does the health gain demonstrated compare with other treatments competing for the NHS's limited resources?

Theory of purchasing

The theory is that any purchaser has a choice about the services it purchases, which is based on information about the cost and effectiveness of these services. The cost of interferon-β is likely to be about £10 000 per patient per year, and the benefits of treatment can be calculated from the published trial,[1] giving a cost of £21 276 per exacerbation prevented or £23 584 per hospital inpatient day prevented. Prevention of hospital admission may not be the most appropriate outcome measure for multiple sclerosis, but it is the only one that can be used to give a comparison between treatments from the published data.

Table 16.1 compares the costs of drugs used in potentially fatal chronic diseases that are currently competing for purchasers' resources and the costs of purchasing these drugs for all patients in North West region who would benefit. Compared with clozapine and dornase α, interferon-β does not seem to be a good buy. If purchasers were making real choices about investment, interferon-β would not be a priority as it would seriously impair their ability to purchase more cost effective treatments.

The reality of purchasing

A group of professional advisers from purchasers in North West region was convened in November 1994 after a notification from the regional drug information service. There was broad agreement that, in light of current evidence, the marginal benefit of the drug did not seem to justify the likely investment.

The working group agreed upon five options for purchasers:

1 Do not fund any prescribing at this stage

2 Limited prescribing through specialist neurology centres only
3 Prescribing by neurologists only within regionally agreed guidelines
4 Shared care with general practitioners—consultants initiate treatment, but GPs prescribe maintenance treatment and absorb costs in primary care prescribing budget
5 Prescribing initiated and maintained by GPs.

Option 1, although rational in view of the above data about cost effectiveness, was not considered to be politically sustainable after discussions with key groups such as the Multiple Sclerosis Society, GPs, and colleagues from the regional health authority and the Department of Health. Option 2 was not considered to be the ideal option because of a concurrent review of neurology services in the region, and the advisory group had no desire to promote any particular service configuration. The advantages and disadvantages of options 3–5 have been discussed by Walley and Barton.[6] Option 3—keeping prescribing within hospitals—had the advantage of making it easier to target the drug appropriately and maintain a universal audit system among all prescribers. Options 4 and 5 were excluded because it was considered that general practitioner prescribing could lead to patients who did not meet the entry criteria of the trial[1] receiving the drug.

However, assessment of patients for the drug would further stretch neurology services, which already had substantial waiting times. An investment in neurology services was needed to avoid GPs being pressured to prescribe. Preliminary estimates of the drug's annual costs for the region varied from £30m (45% of patients with multiple sclerosis receiving the drug) to £0·67m (1% receiving the drug). Option 3 was finally recommended to purchaser chief executives, and a commitment to invest in neurology services was made.

The drug company's marketing strategy involved offering "free" nurses as part of a support package of care. Although current nursing support was felt to be inadequate, there were reservations about accepting product specific nurses because, first, they could encourage consultants to prescribe the drug in order to gain nursing support and, second, there were other products in the pipeline to be considered. Consequently, each hospital was asked to draw up its own profile of service costs that included nursing.

Views of neurologists

Neurologists in the region varied in their opinion of the value of the drug. A preliminary paper from Professor McDonald of the National Hospital for Neurology and Neurosurgery suggested that widespread prescribing of the drug could not yet be justified.[7] Some local neurologists did not wish to prescribe the drug on the basis of current evidence and thought that any additional resources should be directed to better supportive care for patients with multiple sclerosis. Others thought that patients should be able to try any new product that had shown some benefit.

A meeting was arranged with Professor McDonald, who was preparing guidelines for the Association of British Neurologists, to give neurologists in North West region the opportunity to influence these national guidelines and assist in developing some local consensus. Neurologists thought that the assessment of patients should, ideally, be undertaken by neurologists, who were in short supply, although some felt that elements of the assessment could be delegated to other health professionals. If patients with multiple sclerosis were not seen quickly they might pressure their GP to prescribe the drug, and this was not thought to be clinically appropriate. However, there was a danger that this drug could distort clinical priorities. A policy of giving priority to patients with multiple sclerosis over patients with other diagnoses was not acceptable to most doctors.

Communications

Consultation and communication with all the key players were an essential part of the strategy. In view of the high profile of this drug, the NHS Executive was consulted at key stages to ensure that our local actions did not conflict with national policy. Communicating progress to GPs, professional advisers, and managers was time consuming. Communicating with the general public was more difficult—for example, an attempt to provide journalists with unbiased information to avoid sensationalist stories at the time of the drug's launch was abandoned as journalists were reluctant to spend time on a story that could not be published immediately.

Conclusions

Purchasers were unable to decline funding for a marginally effective drug and thereby undertake explicit rationing. To ensure prescribing was within the guidelines, a vast communication network had to be sustained with managers, GPs, neurologists, the Multiple Sclerosis Society, and professional advisers in all the purchasing authorities. The workload involved was considerable.

The impact of this drug on the NHS will be apparent over the next few years. Purchasers fear that, if the guidelines are not tight enough to limit prescribing within available resources or neurologists find themselves unable to stick to them because of patient pressure, then resources will be sucked from elsewhere in the NHS to fund this drug. Neurologists fear that if uptake is greater than predicted then implicit rationing beyond the criteria in the guidelines may be needed, even though purchasers state that they are committed to fund prescribing within the guidelines.

Acknowledgments

We particularly thank all the neurologists in the North West Region, who steadfastly refused to cancel any clinical commitments to talk to us but devoted many evenings and lunchtimes to open and thoughtful discussions without which progress would not have occurred.

1 The IFNB Multiple Sclerosis Study Group. Interferon beta-1b is effective in relapsing-remitting multiple sclerosis. Clinical results of a multi-centre, randomised, double blind placebo controlled trial. *Neurology* 1993;**43**:655-61.
2 Meltzer HY, Cola P, Way L, Thompson PA, Bastani B, Davies MA. Cost effectiveness of clozapine in neuroleptic-resistant schizophrenia. *Am J Psychiatry* 1993;**150**:1630-8.
3 Davies LM, Drummond MF. The economic burden of schizophrenia. *Psychiatr Bull* 1990; **14**:522-5.
4 Fuchs HJ, Borowitz DS, Christiansen DH, Morris EM, Nash ML, Ramsey BW for Pulmozyme Study Group. Effect of aerosolized recombinant human DNAse on exacerbations of respiratory symptoms and on pulmonary function in patients with cystic fibrosis. *N Engl J Med* 1994;**331**:637-42.
5 Elborn JS, Shale D, Britton JR. Cystic fibrosis: current survival and population estimates to the year 2000. *Thorax* 1991;**46**:881-5.
6 Walley T, Barton S. A purchaser perspective of managing new drugs: interferon beta as a case study. *BMJ* 1995;**311**:796-9.
7 McDonald WI. New treatments for multiple sclerosis [editorial]. *BMJ* 1995;**310**:345-6.

17 How can hospitals ration drugs?

Drug rationing in a teaching hospital: a method to assign priorities

FELIX BOCHNER, E DEAN MARTIN, NAOMI G BURGESS, ANDREW A SOMOGYI, GARY MH MISAN on behalf of the Drug Committee of the Royal Adelaide Hospital

The cost of all aspects of health care in developed countries is increasing at an alarming rate.[1] Meeting these costs is becoming more difficult, and a variety of cost containment measures is being considered at national and regional levels.[2,3] The continuing introduction of new technologies and drugs is one of the factors in the escalating cost of health care. These new treatments are often incompletely evaluated, and estimates of cost–benefit are lacking or poorly documented. This situation has resulted in a vigorous debate about the need for, ethics of, and possible methods for cost containment and rationing of health services.[4-8]

Hospitals have responded to shrinking financial resources by: increasing day patient or outpatient services; transferring outpatient services to the community; imposing waiting lists; making services available only as long as funds are available; and withdrawing some services altogether. The last two options, and to some extent the imposition of waiting lists, are usually unplanned because cuts in hospital or divisional budgets often occur with little warning, and they can be regarded as arbitrary and unfair. Those patients who are excluded from the curtailed or reduced service are often those who were the last to join the queue.

The Royal Adelaide Hospital is a tertiary referral hospital of about 900 beds. The annual allocation for drugs is 4·6% of total expenditure and has remained more or less fixed since 1988, when the administrators decreed that expenditure on drugs was not to exceed this allocation. The

237

Table 17.1   Unfunded initiatives, in alphabetical order, and their projected cost and indications in the 1992–3 financial year.

Drug	Indication	Cost ($A)
Antithymocyte globulin	Aplastic anaemia	32 000
Botulinum A toxin	Dystonias	10 000
Budesonide turbohaler	Asthma	4000
Carboplatin	Neoplasms (general use)	45 000
	CIS–Platinum contraindicated	3000
Desmopressin	Postoperative bleeding	
	(cardiothoracic surgery)	108 000
Fluconazole	Fungal infection	40 000
Fluoxetine	Depression	10 000
Low molecular weight	Hip replacement	15 000
heparin	Haemodialysis	30 000
Interferon	Chronic myeloid leukaemia	240 000
	Hairy cell leukaemia	12 000
	Hepatitis C	56 000
	Hepatatis B	30 400
Midazolam	Endoscopy	5000
Morphine slow release	Cancer pain	100 000
Octreotide	Acromegaly	68 000
Ondansetron	Emesis induced by chemotherapy	16 000
Oxpentifylline	Bone marrow transplantation	2 850
Total		730 050

hospital's drug committee introduced several strategies to deal with what was essentially a reduction in its allocation, given that it had to continue to satisfy the demand for new drugs. These measures included continuing the formulary system, some administrative changes, and implementing an ongoing drug utilisation review programme.[9] These measures were reasonably successful until the middle of 1991, when it became apparent that unless additional funds were made available it would be impossible to introduce new drugs or new indications for existing drugs. Since additional money was not available, all requests for new therapeutic initiatives, which by this time were considerable (Table 17.1) and would have cost an additional $730 000 annually (just under 10% of the drug budget), were refused until funds could be liberated from other sources. The drug committee was therefore faced with the dilemma of which new drugs to include in the formulary if additional funds became available.

A method (to be called the funding model) to assign ranking priorities by means of a formal scoring system was used for previously unfunded initiatives to allow their serial and orderly introduction into the hospital formulary. We report our experience and the initial responses from the hospital staff to an activity that was, in essence, overt and explicit rationing.

238

Methods

The Drug Committee

The Drug Committee must ensure that drug availability and prescribing in the Royal Adelaide Hospital conforms to the highest contemporary standards. The Committee is composed of nine elected members representing clinicians (two physicians, two surgeons, one haematologist, one radiotherapist, one clinical pharmacologist, one occupational physician, one nurse) and four *ex officio* members representing the pharmacy department (two), the medical administration (one), and the finance department. The Committee is thus composed predominantly of people involved in patient care and regular drug prescribing.

Several steps take place before the final inclusion (or otherwise) of a drug in the hospital's formulary. These are application from members of the consultant staff for a drug; development of treatment and usage guidelines by the relevant experts (almost always drawn from the hospital's staff); consideration by the Committee of the request and its guidelines; the decision to accept or reject the application, based on clinical and scientific grounds; and evaluation of the financial impact of inclusion of the drug into the formulary.

The ranking model

Principles

The ranking model was based on six principles. First, a treatment should be based on careful deliberation of clinical, professional, scientific and health economic considerations and should not be dominated by cost factors alone. Second, protocols and treatment guidelines should be established for all drug treatments at the hospital (this principle presumes that such protocols or guidelines will lead to improved standards of patient care and would form the basis for clinical education, future medical audits, or drug utilisation reviews). Third, protocol and treatment guidelines should be explicit and should clearly define how the experts believe the new drug should be used in the hospital in relation to all of the elements described in Box 1. Fourth, a request for inclusion into the formulary and subsequent ranking by the model would proceed only if the drug qualified on clinical and scientific grounds based on the criteria in the box. Fifth, the use of investigational therapies such as new drugs or established drugs for new indications or in new protocols (after appropriate ethical review) should not be discouraged. Sixth, priorities in allocating resources for all treatments

239

Box 1—Information required for drug inclusion into formulary

- Description of new treatment
- Treatment indications
- Patient selection (inclusion and exclusion) criteria
- Treatment objective
- First, second, and other treatment options
- Precise treatment end points
- Drug dosage and schedule (including duration of treatment)
- Anticipated annual patient numbers
- Safety and efficacy considerations (including comparisons with other treatments)
- Financial considerations including comparisons of cost differentials with other treatment options (including non-drug options)

---

should be determined by the hospital's clinicians and by multidisciplinary consultation.

At an operational level, the guiding principles were that the ranking of drug requests is based on the need to obtain the greatest benefit for the most patients for each dollar spent[10] and that the ranking model takes into account the quality and cost of the treatment and must be sufficiently robust to minimise subjectivity and enhance consistency in decision making. Thus the ranking model should enable the hospital (through its Drug Committee) to decide whether to fund, for example, ondansetron for an estimated 55 patients annually at a cost of A$16 000 or midazolam for an estimated 4000 patients at an annual cost of A$5000. The model was modified several times before it was considered suitable for application. The version in current use is described.

Calculation of score value to assign ordered ranking

The final score (or ratio) has two components. The numerator consists of a quality score and the denominator of a cost score. The process of determining the score is summarised in Box 2.

The quality score has three elements. The first is the outcome score. For individual patient benefit, values are assigned as follows: if the drug results in cure (for example, fluconazole for fungal infection) or is used for prophylaxis (low molecular weight heparin in hip replacement) the value is 30; if the drug prolongs life, the value is 15; if it causes palliation or symptom control, it achieves a value of 7; and if it is no better than placebo, it is assigned a score of 0. Mortality/morbidity of the disease or condition for which the drug is indicated attracts scores as follows: 9/5, 6/3, and

240

Box 2—Derivation of final ratio score

Quality score

1 *Outcome*
  1.1 Patient benefit
  - Cure/prevention (30)
  - Prolongation of life (15)
  - Palliation/symptom control (7)
  - Placebo (0)
  1.2 Mortality/morbidity
  - High risk (9/5)
  - Moderate risk (6/3)
  - Low risk (3/1)
  1.3 Response
  - Expected response rate based on the scientific literature
  Outcome score $= (1 \cdot 1 + 1 \cdot 2) \times 1 \cdot 3$

2 *Type of treatment*
  - Established indication (5)
  - New therapy (3)
  - Trial/investigational (1)

3 *Clinical comparison with other treatments*
  - No alternative (15)
  - New treatment >existing (10)
  - New treatment = existing (5)
  - Existing treatment >new (0)

Final quality score = outcome + treatment type + clinical comparison

Cost score

Comparison with other treatments
  - New treatment less expensive (0)
  - No alternative (2)
  - New treatment = existing (5)
  - New treatment more expensive (10)
  Total cost per year (in $7500 increments) (1-7)
  Cost per patient (in $750 increments) (1-7)

Final cost score = cost comparison + total cost per year + cost per patient

Final ratio = total quality score/total cost score

- The higher the ratio, the higher the priority to provide funds

3/1 for conditions of high (>75%), moderate (35–75%) or low (<35%) mortality/morbidity respectively (mortality score relates only to the cure/ prevention outcome). The third component is response: for example, if the treatment results in an average 90% cure rate the assigned value is 0·9. The score is calculated as the sum of the scores obtained from the individual patient benefit and mortality/morbidity categories multiplied by the response score.

The second element is the type of treatment. A score of 5 is allocated for an indication that is well established or for which the drug has proved effectiveness; 3 if it is a new treatment; and 1 if it is a trial or investigational drug.

The third element is the clinical comparison with other treatments available and takes into account such factors as efficacy, adverse effects, attributes that may affect patient compliance, and ease with which the drug can be given to patients. Scores of 15 are assigned if there is no alternative to the new treatment; 10 if the new treatment is better than existing treatment; 5 if the treatment equals existing treatment; and zero if the existing treatment is better than the new treatment.

The final quality score is the sum of the scores obtained from the outcome, type of treatment and clinical comparison scores. An example of how this can be derived is shown in Box 3.

Box 3—Example of how various elements of numerator and denominator were derived to obtain final score

Fluconazole

Indication: cryptococcal meningitis where amphotericin is contraindicated
Outcome score:
   Cure of disease of high mortality with 85% response rate =
$(30 + 9) \times 0·85 = 33·15$
Quality score:
   Outcome (33·15) + established effectiveness (5) + new treatment existing (10) = 48·15
Cost score:
   Cost per patient: A$750–100
   Number of patients per year: 35
   Total cost per year: A$40 000–A$45 000
No alternative treatment (2) + A$40 000–A$45 000 annually (6) + A$750–A$1500 per patient (2) = 10
Final ratio: 48·15–10 = 4·8

The cost score also contains three elements. The first is the cost comparison with alternative or existing treatments. Scores of 0 are allocated if the new treatment is less expensive than existing treatment; 2 if there is no alternative to the new drug; 5 if the new drug cost equals the cost of existing treatment, and 10 if the new treatment is more expensive than currently available treatments.

The second element is the total cost per year for the newly introduced drug at the Royal Adelaide Hospital. This cost is based on the cost of the drug multiplied by the total number of patients who qualify for the drug. Scores ranging from 1 to 7 are allocated for each of seven bands, with each band equating to A$7500. For example, a score of 1 is assigned for a drug costing less than A$7500 annually, 6 for a cost of A$37 500 to A$45 000 annually, and 7 for a drug costing more than A$45 000 annually. Higher scores for a greater annual cost beyond A$45 000 are not assigned, because this would result in cost and not clinical considerations becoming the dominant factor in arriving at the ranking score. The cost used is the marginal or incremental cost resulting from replacing an existing treatment with a new one. If no new treatment is being replaced, the marginal cost equals total new drug cost. This provides a measure of the additional impact on the total drug budget.

The third element is the cost per individual patient for a completed treatment course. Here also scores ranging from 1 to 7 were allocated for each of seven bands, with each band representing A$750. A treatment costing less than $A750 was assigned a score of 1, and one costing more than $A4500 a score of 7. For the same reasons as given above, a score higher than 7 was not assigned if the treatment cost exceeded A$4500.

The final cost score is the sum of the scores obtained from the three elements just described. All costs are expressed in Australian dollars. Box 3 contains an example of how the cost score was derived.

The final ratio score is calculated as the quality score divided by the cost score (see Box 3 for example).

Results

The quality, cost, and ratio scores and the final ranking of the 19 unfunded initiatives (alphabetically listed in Table 17.1) are shown in Table 17.2. The ranking can be used to allocate available resources in order of the priority. Additional resources became available in June 1992 (coinciding with the end of the Australian financial year) to fund the first 11 initiatives in Table 17.2, and these were introduced into the hospital's formulary. The version of the model reported here evolved from several earlier versions, none of which produced ratio scores that discriminated sufficiently between drugs. The model has been widely disseminated and debated by the hospital staff. At the time of writing this report, there was general agreement that demand for services was outstripping the available resources; that some

Table 17.2   Final ranking of the 19 unfunded initiatives, giving the numerator (quality), denominator (cost), and final ratio scores

Priority No.	Drug	Quality score	Cost score	Ratio score
1	Oxypentifylline	25·2	2	12·6
2	Interferon (hairy cell leukaemia)	52·4	10	5·2
3	Fluconazole	48·2	10	4·8
4	Botulinum A toxin	22·2	5	4·4
5	Low molecular weight heparin (hip replacement)	41·4	13	3·2
6	Budesonide turbohaler	31·2	12	2·6
7	Interferon (hepatitis C)	29·0	12	2·4
8	Low molecular weight heparin (haemodialysis)	36·4	16	2·3
8	Interferon (hepatitis B)	32.6	14	2·3
8	Antithymocyte globulin	38·4	17	2·3
11	Octreotide	36·0	16	2·3
12	Carboplatin (cisplatin contraindicated)	22·5	12	1·9
13	Ondansetron	25·8	14	1·8
14	Interferon (chronic myeloid leukaemia)	27·2	16	1·7
15	Desmopressin	20·0	13	1·5
15	Midazolam	18·0	12	1·5
17	Morphine slow release	24·9	19	1·3
17	Fluoxetine	17·0	13	1·3
19	Carboplatin (general use)	17·5	19	0·9

measures were needed to remedy the immediate situation; that the principles on which the model was based were appropriate; that a model such as this one, although simplistic, deserved a trial; and that the ethics of resource rationing needed close scrutiny and debate in the hospital and, equally importantly, in the community.

Discussion

Most teaching hospitals are likely to be faced with the dilemma of shrinking resources. One solution is to obtain increased funding; another is to impose measures to enable targeting of available resources to activities that are considered to be the most cost effective. As the first option is becoming increasingly difficult to achieve, and in the view of some[8 11] to justify, this realistically leaves only the second option if teaching hospitals are to continue their traditional roles. The imperative to improve methods by which allocation and rationing decisions are made has been enunciated for at least a decade in the context of national and regional health delivery programmes.[1,5,10,12-17] Thus the development of this model can be seen as occurring in a climate of acceptance, albeit reluctant, of the need to consider

244

rationing. The decision to create a model for more equitable and transparent means to distribute drugs was driven by the administration's mandate for a balanced drug budget, akin to the situation described for the state of Oregon.[14]

The introduction of the ranking model was underpinned by some important principles, which had already been accepted by the hospital's staff. The first is that provision of services must be based on the best currently available scientific evidence. The adoption of the criteria in Box 1 has led to a far more critical appraisal of the potential of a drug or treatment. Unless a drug was considered satisfactory by these criteria, it was rejected for inclusion in the formulary, even if the cost was minimal. Second, these criteria are central to the hospital's ongoing drug utilisation review programme, which has resulted in increased awareness of the need for frequent re-evaluation of current practices, improved patient care, and, coincidentally, cost savings.[9] Third, although calculation of the ranking score ratio was initially based on the principles of cost effectiveness analysis,[18-21] cost was not allowed to dominate the final result, because this would have denied certain patient groups potentially life saving but expensive treatments and would have been contrary to the "rule of rescue", which dictates that there is a perceived duty to save endangered life where possible. A similar circumstance occurred when the planners in Oregon had to modify the initial list of priorities to raise certain life threatening conditions above less important ones.[20,22-23] It would have proved difficult, if not impossible, to obtain the agreement of the clinicians on the Drug Committee and the hospital to proceed with the development and implementation of the ranking model if cost had dominated the final outcome. This observation is in accord with the contention that "a rational plan needs to have medical and ethical, not simply economic, justification".[24]

Any model that reduces matters of life, death, or morbidity to a numerical value must be simple to use and must be clinically relevant if it is to find acceptance. Whether our model satisfies these requirements will depend on several of the "input" variables. Are the patient outcome data robust?[25] How can degrees of morbidity or suffering be measured and how can these subjective variables be compared across different patients and disease states (see below)? How reliable are estimates of numbers of patients needing the new treatments? The Committee acknowledged that even the best available evidence was often incomplete or inconclusive. Despite these deficiencies and the relative simplicity of the model, it was felt that the experiment was worth pursuing, rather than continuing to apply arbitrary and sometimes arguably unfair decisions to drug availability. The fact that the hospital community has so far accepted ranking decisions which have resulted from application of the model suggests that there is some clinical validity to the process. The final scores were obtained from data which for the denominator were specific to the drug budget of the Royal Adelaide

Hospital. There is no reason why the model could not be transportable to other institutions, and possibly even to other areas of healthcare delivery and resource planning. The only requirement is that the information that is incorporated into the model should be scientifically sound and be relevant to the setting in which it is to be used.

Comparing subjective variables

There was considerable debate about how to estimate and compare potential benefits to patients with different conditions of differing severity for which different treatments were indicated. The Committee wished to have a method that would be as precise as possible, because the quality score (numerator) incorporates elements of patient outcome in each of the three components. Incorrect assessment of outcome in a pessimistic or optimistic direction could substantially distort the numerator score and render the model useless. The data used in the denominator were considered to be less subjective and more easily quantifiable. We rejected the use of the quality adjusted life year (QALY) as an outcome measure for three reasons: explicit QALY information for most drug outcomes is not yet available; assigning a QALY to a drug intervention is likely to be as subjective and potentially inaccurate[26] as the method currently used, because assessment of quality of years must be embedded in a knowledge of the likely disease process[10,26] and this could be highly variable from patient to patient; and there are interventions for which QALYs are difficult to measure, especially those that reduce short term disabilities such as nausea or vomiting and pain.[27]

The probabilities assumptions about effectiveness and outcomes were taken from the best published evidence and extrapolated to apply to the patient population in our hospital. The final weightings we applied to the various categories in the numerator were arbitrary but were based on the principle that a treatment that resulted in cure or prevention of a condition with high mortality should be accorded a higher score than one that was only palliative. This is reflected in the approximate doubling of the relative weightings between each category in the individual patient benefit scores and the deliberate overlap between mortality and morbidity scores.

Questions about rationing

Medical practitioners will always feel uncomfortable when faced with a decision that may deny an individual patient a potential benefit. Thus, rationing brings into sharp focus the conflict between a practitioner's responsibility to the individual and to the society in which we live.[19,28-29] Given that covert rationing has been in force in most if not all societies, should rationing decisions be more explicit, and who should participate in the debate that leads to the final decisions about which services will be provided, reduced, or removed? There is a strong argument that the decision making process should be made more open, transparent, and explicit.[1,3,11,26,30,31] Our hospital community was widely consulted about the need for and proposed methods to achieve the ranking model described here. There were inevitably arguments of competing priorities, but decisions arising from application of the ranking model have so far been accepted.

Who should arbitrate about what is to be rationed? There are four interested parties to consider: politicians (the idealogues), administrators (the health funders), clinicians (health deliverers), and patients (health recipients). In this instance, the administrators issued the mandate not to exceed budgetary allocations, thus implicitly imposing rationing decisions on the clinicians. This can be defended[31,32] because it is the clinician who has day to day contact with the patient and who is in the best position to be able to arrive at such decisions. A contrary view has been put by Leeder and by Sulmasy, who contended that clinicians should not have to act as restrictive gatekeepers.[33,34] These opposing views were strongly represented among the hospital's staff, but there was a final consensus that clinicians must take part in such a process.

Where does this leave the patient? It has been started that rationing should not be the exclusive domain of managers and professionals,[35,36] because it is the patient who is the final beneficiary (or otherwise) of such decisions. In the long run, rationing by patient choice[35] seems not only logical, but equitable. Substantial methodological issues must be considered, however, before such a situation can become a reality.[35] We did not involve patients nor their representatives in the development of this model. It is hoped that debate generated by the introduction of the model will flow on to the community served by the hospital, and thus enlist the recipients and politicians in crucial decision making processes on the delivery of health care.

Finally, is the model and its application fair? The answer to this lies partly in whether rationing can be considered as fair. It has been stated that "unfairness lies also in doing things until the money runs out"[11] and that "rationing becomes a morally acceptable option if the need is great enough and if other methods have been exhausted".[33] In our case the need had become acute, other methods were not sufficient to meet our requirements, and we could not wait for the ultimate cost saving benefits of the drug utilisation review programme to take effect. A method was therefore needed to provide a more equitable approach to this decision making process.

Acknowledgments

We thank Drs R C A Bartholomeusz and R Kelly for help during the developmental stages of the model. The members of the drug committee during the period described in this report (mid 1991 to end 1992) were: Dr R Antic, Dr C Barker, Dr W Cobain, Mr P Devitt, Mr F Erdt, Dr N Horvath, Mr T I Lee, Dr L Leleu, Ms L Maguire, Mr J A R Williams, and Dr E Yeoh.

1 Heginbotham C. Rationing. *BMJ* 1992;**304**:496–9.
2 Schwartz WB, Aaron HJ. Rationing hospital care. Lessons from Britain. *N Engl J Med* 1984;**310**:52–6.
3 Dixon J, Welch HG. Priority setting: lessons from Oregon. *Lancet* 1991;**337**:891–4.
4 Fuchs VR. The "rationing" of medical care. *N Engl J Med* 1984;**311**:1572–3.
5 Leaf A. The doctor's dilemma—and society's too. *N Engl J Med* 1984;**310**:718–21.
6 Daniels N. Why saying no to patients in the United States is so hard. Cost containment, justice, and provider autonomy. *N Engl J Med* 1986;**314**:1380–3.
7 Relman AS. Is rationing inevitable? *N Engl J Med* 1990;**322**:1809–10.
8 Callahan D. Rationing medical progress. The way to affordable health care. *N Engl J Med* 1990;**322**:1810–3.
9 Misan GMH, Martin ED, Smith ER, Somogyi AA, Bartholomeusz RCA, Bochner F. Drug utilisation review in a teaching hospital: experience with vancomycin. *Eur J Clin Pharmacol* 1990;**39**:457–61.
10 Normand C. Economics, health, and the economics of health. *BMF* 1991;**303**:1572–7.
11 Leeder SR. All for one or one for all? The ethics of resource allocation for health care. *Med J Aust* 1987;**147**:68–71.
12 Evans RW. Health care technology and the inevitability of resource allocation and rationing decisions. Part I. *JAMA* 1983;**249**:2047–53.
13 Evans RW. Health care technology and the inevitability of resource allocation and rationing decisions. Part II. *JAMA* 1983;**249**:2208–19.
14 Welch HG, Larson E. Dealing with limited resources. The Oregon decision to curtail funding for organ transplantation. *N Engl J Med* 1988;**319**:171–3.
15 Lewis PA, Charny M. Which of two individuals do you treat when only their ages are different and you can't treat both? *J Med Ethics* 1989;**15**:28–32.
16 Lamb D. Priorities in health care: reply to Lewis and Charny. *J Med Ethics* 1989;**15**:33–4.
17 Larkins R. Patient care when medical resources are scarce. *Australian Medicine* 1989;**1**:377–9.
18 Beck JR. How to evaluate drugs. Cost-effectiveness analysis. *FAMA* 1990;**264**:83–4.
19 Detsky AS, Naglie IG. A clinician's guide to cost–effectiveness analysis. *Ann Intern Med* 1990;**113**:147–54.
20 Eddy DM. Oregon's methods. Did cost-effectiveness analysis fail? *JAMA* 1991;**266**:2135–41.
21 Eddy DM. Cost-effectiveness analysis. A conversation with my father. *JAMA* 1992;**267**:1669–75.
22 Hadorn DC. Setting health priorities in Oregon. Cost effectiveness meets the rule of rescue. *JAMA* 1991;**265**:2218–25.
23 Eddy DM. Oregon's plan. Should it be approved? *JAMA* 1991;**266**:2439–45.
24 Relman AS. The trouble with rationing. *N Engl J Med* 1990;**323**:911–3.
25 Eddy DM. Cost-effectiveness analysis. Is it up to the task? *JAMA* 1992;**267**:3342–8.
26 Klein R. On the Oregon trail: rationing health care. More politics than science. *BMJ* 1991;**302**:1–2.
27 Laupacis A, Feeny D, Detsky AS, Tugwell PX. How attractive does a new technology have to be to warrant adoption and utilisation? Tentative guidelines for using clinical and economic evaluations. *Can Med Assoc J* 1992;**146**:473–81.
28 Eddy DM. The individual vs society. Is there a conflict? *JAMA* 1991;**265**:1446–50.

29 Eddy DM. The individual vs society. Resolving the conflict. *JAMA* 1991;**265**:2399–406.
30 Eddy DM. Practice policies—guidelines for methods. *JAMA* 1990;**263**:1839–41.
31 Smith R. Rationing: the search for sunlight. Rationing decisions should be explicit and rational. *BMJ* 1991;**303**:1561–2.
32 Klein R. Warning signals from Oregon. The different dimensions of rationing need untangling. *BMJ* 1992;**304**:1457–8.
33 Leeder SR. Cost cutting without blood spilling. *Hospital and Healthcare Australia* 1989; **20**(Nov):16,18,30.
34 Sulmasy DP. Physicians, cost control, and ethics. *Ann Intern Med* 1992;**116**:920–6.
35 Eddy DM. Rationing by patient choice. *JAMA* 1991;**265**:105–8.
36 Chaturvedi N. Rationing. *BMJ* 1993;**306**:395.

Formulate, don't formularise

CAM DONALDSON

Too often decisions about the allocation of scarce resources are being formularised (that is, crammed into formulae) rather than formulated (structured on the basis of thought). Those who use the formula of Bochner *et al* uncritically will be guilty of this. Many users of economic criteria, such as QALY league tables, also fall into this trap. The aim of this commentary is to outline, from an economic perspective, why this is a problem and what can be done about it.

Formularising hides subjectivity . . .

Clinicians and pharmacists are hard people. They are taught to think that subjectivity is "woolly". This leads to a desire to quantify all relevant considerations in a formula in the belief that this somehow makes things objective. This quantification goes on regardless of whether the elements of the formula overlap (as they do in the case of Bochner *et al*) and of whether it is in fact theoretically or practically relevant to combine these elements in the way formulae do. There is a failure to recognise that all resource allocation is (and must be) based on subjectivity, whether or not a formula is used. The will-o'-the-wisp pursuit of objectivity through formulae hides this fact in a way which is unhelpful.

249

... so let's formulate ...

Without clear thinking, formulae can be constructed on arbitrary bases. In such cases decision making will not be improved. Less effort should go into fine tuning the elements of formulae and more into thinking about what their devisers were trying to achieve in the first place. In this regard, unmasking some of the arbitrary and subjective constructs of the formula of Bochner *et al* can help us discard some of the elements it contains. For instance:

- Is a cure for a high risk condition causing morbidity (with a score of 150) worth more than prolongation of life for a moderate risk condition (with score of 90)? (The formula says "Yes"; I say "probably not"; what does the reader think?)
- Of two new drugs that are otherwise equivalent, is drug A of higher priority than drug B because B's total costs are greater? (The formula says "Yes"; I say "No"; what does the reader think?)

In the first case too much emphasis is placed on "risk" and on "curing". In the second case, drug B may marginally increase costs over its already expensive alternative, while drug A could increase costs tenfold over its cheap alternative and still be valued higher than B. Total cost is distorting the result when it should not be counted at all. In both cases, progress can be made by thinking about the problem and formulating it in terms of relevant criteria for maximising benefits for resources spent.

... and get our objectives sorted out

Although it is not clear, I think the authors are concerned with maximising benefits to patients with existing resources. If so, all that matters is whether the benefit per pound spent on treating a patient with condition X is greater or less than that for treating a patient with condition Y. If the returns from treating X are greater than for treating Y, some resources should be moved out of treating Ys and into treating Xs. If a new drug becomes available to treat condition Y, the next question is whether the situation is altered. The only factors relevant to this from the Bochner *et al* formula are a reformulated version of the quality score (dropping the mortality/morbidity component) and some combination of two components of the cost score, the comparison with other treatments and the total cost per year. The quality of the information, as reflected in type of treatment, matters but only in so far as whether or not to defer a decision. To quantify the quality of information and add to it outcome before dividing by cost has no theoretical or practical justification. It is adding the "unaddable" and dividing the indivisible.

Conclusion

Purchasers and providers of health care everywhere need to recognise that, because of a lack of data, and even with good data, priority setting is about making judgments. Formulas based on arbitrary constructs, such as that of Bochner *et al* do not improve such decision making. In a complex world, economics is better used to help provide a framework for such judgments rather than as justification for the "quick fix" of formulae. Purchasers in particular need to grasp this nettle. Otherwise, services will continue to be provider dominated.

Health economists and health care professionals need to get together on these issues. They will then benefit from each other's skills, rather than each group developing formulae for the other group to criticise. As long as the twain never meet then neither of the twain shall have relevance to priority setting for maximum health gain to the community.

First consider the overall process of care

J C PETRIE

The description of Bochner *et al*'s method deserves critical scrutiny as the subject of drug rationing raises important issues. The argument to ration drugs is based on the wish to obtain the greatest benefit for most patients for each dollar spent on drugs. This premise requires rigorous examination before local drug rationing is applied. Have the authors ensured that they have obtained full value for the money that they spend on drugs and on care services before implementing their rationing policy for drugs? In some health services, for each £100 spent on drugs as little as 15% of value may be obtained.

The price of individual drug entities is only one factor—and a minor factor—in the overall costs of the process of care. Should health professionals not act as advocates to ensure that essential drugs of an acceptable quality and quantity are available within the overall resources available? This approach requires the development and monitoring of guidelines and local care protocols of affordable quality for the management and appropriate

251

follow up of specific diseases to get full value for the money spent. Team work (including substitution), drug formularies, and the effective selection, procurement, and utilisation of drugs by informed health professionals have much potential to release resources that may be directed to purchase, and not ration, drugs.

In my opinion drug rationing should only be imposed if it has been clearly established that within the resources available for all health purposes the cost effective delivery of other aspects of care has been ensured. If rationing of drugs is to be implemented and individual patients denied potentially life saving expensive drugs, this health policy should be explicitly made known and debated with the public and (in the UK) with the purchasers. Are patients admitted to the Adelaide hospital aware that they are subject to drug rationing, and of the criteria? Can they choose to be admitted to another hospital in Adelaide? Is there informed consent? What is the legal position of the local managers, of the drug and therapeutic (medicines) committees, and of its members?

The issue is even more complicated. For example, the pharmacoeconomic arguments are complex. Neither patients, their families, other local hospitals—general or private—nor local practitioners seem to have been involved in the decisions to ration drugs. Uncritical acceptance and application of the principles behind the local judgments could lead to direct harm to individual patients.

The methodology to derive the scoring system also has to be carefully assessed and validated. Has the objectivity and reproducibility of this funding or ranking method been evaluated? The authors describe continuing change in the model. They concede that the cost factor becomes very difficult to manage at a particular point. As this is the biggest problem in finding new money for new drugs, it poses a real problem for the model. Judgmental scoring systems, which have a qualitative element, are notoriously difficult to validate and interpret. Different observers value items differently. What evidence is there that the Adelaide expertise is reproducible, standardised, and objective? The authors face the problem of measuring quality in numerical mode, and manipulating judgmental pseudonumbers to reach debatable conclusions. They have not shown evidence of a clearly objective score. Nor have they produced results of the outcomes (mortality, quality, patient views, costs, present state of the formulary) of their policy.

In summary, I have difficulty with the premise of drug rationing in the absence of assurances that the services were otherwise well organised, appropriate, and in place. The ethical and legal implications of the moratorium on spending on drugs imposed by the management require further debate. I believe that there are problems with the present state of the methodology, in particular the strengths and weaknesses of potential approaches to qualitative and quantitative scoring systems and the

252

pharmacoeconomic arguments. Any decision to ration drugs is one that society must make through elected representatives as choices have to be made. The decisions depend on expert advice. I am not confident of the rationale for rationing in Adelaide nor of the robustness of the "Adelaide model" as described.

Fairness is at issue

RUTH CHADWICK

The last paragraph of Bochner *et al's* paper asks whether the model and its application are fair. The answer is said to depend on whether rationing itself is fair. And yet arguably the very concept of rationing (as in postwar rationing, for example) involves sharing resources equitably, giving each person their portion. How to achieve an equitable distribution is the issue. In the current debates about allocation of healthcare resources, however, the term "rationing" has acquired a bad image, whereas "priority setting" has for some reason been thought preferable, although setting priorities precisely does mean giving preference to some areas and thus some people, with the implication that others will go without.

The model outlined is one that gives priority to some drugs over others—some will not fall within the budget at all. Is this fair? The question turns on what criteria of allocation are used. A procedural requirement of fairness is that like cases are treated alike: the authors admit the desirability of consistency in decision making. There is a question, however, as to whether consistency in treatment of drugs is what is desirable, rather than consistency in treatment of people. Although it is claimed that cost was not allowed to override other considerations to the extent that certain patient groups would be denied potentially life saving though expensive treatment, the system proposed will surely have this effect at times: some people will not receive what they need. Concentration on choosing between drugs distances the decision makers from this fact.

There are strong, though not universally accepted, arguments for the view that distributing resources according to need is what is fair. In Bochner *et al's* paper, however, the first guiding principle at an operational level is based on the "need to obtain the greatest benefit for the most patients for each dollar spent". In what sense this is a "need" is not made clear. Further,

253

as in the case of the utilitarian principle of maximising the greatest happiness for the greatest number, this looks like one principle but in fact contains two parts: "greatest benefit" and "most patients". The fact that these can conflict is disguised by the example of a choice between 55 patients at A$16 000 and 4000 at A$5000. What if the choice is between 55 and 4000 for the same cost, where the 55 gain a much greater benefit than the 4000? This presents starkly the clash between "greatest benefit" to a few and the smaller benefit to "most patients".

This issue gives rise to the problem, recognised by the authors, of the difficult issues surrounding interpersonal comparisons, which of course affect most if not all criteria of allocation. Measurement by QALY is rejected partly on the ground that it is "likely to be as subjective and potentially inaccurate as the method currently used". This hardly seems a strong argument for preferring the latter. Intuition is appealed to as a rationale for according a score of 30 to a treatment that results in cure or prevention of an undesirable outcome while one that prolongs life receives 15. There are several problems here. First, what is meant by "cure" and "undesirable outcome"? How is cure distinguished from prolonged life? Even if cure is preferable, is it twice as good?

Some aspects of the description of the model give cause for concern. For example, it is said that there is a tendency to underestimate the number of patients "worthy" of a new treatment. What does "worthy" mean in this context? Finally, the list of interested parties to consider includes patients but does not include society, or the public, who surely have an interest in how healthcare resources are allocated and arguably should have a voice in decisions on criteria of allocation.

Authors' response

We have the impression that our commentators are theorists and have not had the responsibility of managing a capped drug budget in a climate which rightly demands the introduction of new—and often very expensive—drugs. Perhaps they failed to appreciate that the model is only one of several strategies to improve drug use; it was developed to respond to our hospital's restrictions on the drug budget, with the consequent need to impose some rationing to avert an even greater crisis than might have otherwise occurred. This was not some theoretical game, the playing of which involved the luxury of prolonged debate, philosophical meanderings, and testing several economic models.

Cam Donaldson has accused us of creating a formula that lacked clear thought. The elements in our equation were based on the information in Table 17.2 which we believe contains key concepts to allow a judgment to be made about setting priorities for drugs—and for the patients needing them. Some elements of this information are more objective and therefore more easily quantified than other inevitably more subjective elements, but the best available contemporary evidence is used to decide on the allocation of scores, especially in the numerator. We must emphasise that the scores have no inherent value apart from facilitating ranking of requests. Thus, rather than hiding subjectivity, the equation imposes a rigour in the decision making process. At least our clinicians now understand the reasoning behind the final decisions, and actively participate in them. Does Cam Donaldson seriously suggest that total cost should not be counted at all? This statement ignores the reality of the world in which some of us have to function. We agree that priority setting is about making judgments. This model has facilitated the process in our hospital.

Ruth Chadwick echoes many of the concerns we had during the model's gestation. Although the model concentrates on drugs, it equally takes into account the treatment of people and treatment outcomes (see Table 17.2, especially items 2–9). She suggests that the model will deny potentially lifesaving drugs on cost grounds. The introduction of the model has had the opposite effect because this was already happening in our hospital. We accept that the guiding principle behind the model contains two parts. However, the model would accommodate the example cited by Ruth Chadwick, because it is likely that the score generated from the greater benefit experienced by the smaller number of patients would offset the score in the reverse situation. We agree that the word "worthy" carries judgmental overtones; in this context it means those patients who qualify according to the criteria in Table 17.2.

We agree with much of Petrie's commentary. The drug committee sees itself very much as an advocate for the patient and prescriber. The introduction of the model has facilitated rather than hindered the introduction of expensive drugs in our hospital. Other measures (the formulary, generic prescribing, purchase contracts, appropriate management practices, drug utilisation review programme) continue to be aggressively pursued to ensure the best value for money. These were not enough, however, to accommodate all requests for new drugs. We concede

255

that the model has not been formally validated, but it is being used successfully in several other Australian hospitals. The legal implications are real ones and will need to be addressed by individual institutions, but they are not different in principle from the problems arising from imposing waiting lists (probably universally practised and accepted as a "fact of life"), which can result in substantial suffering and even death.

Index